Wild Magic

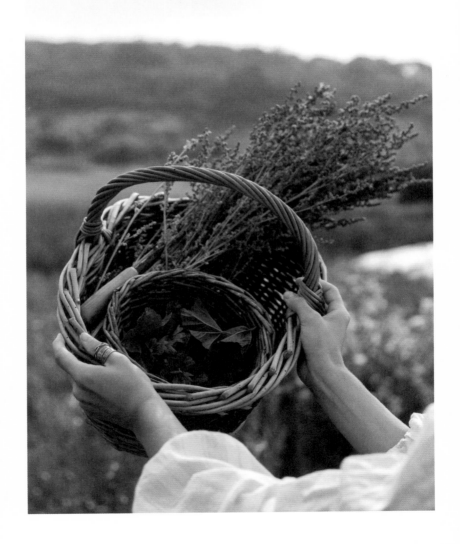

Fern Freud

Wild Magic

A seasonal guide to foraging with healing recipes and self-care rituals

EBURY
PRESS

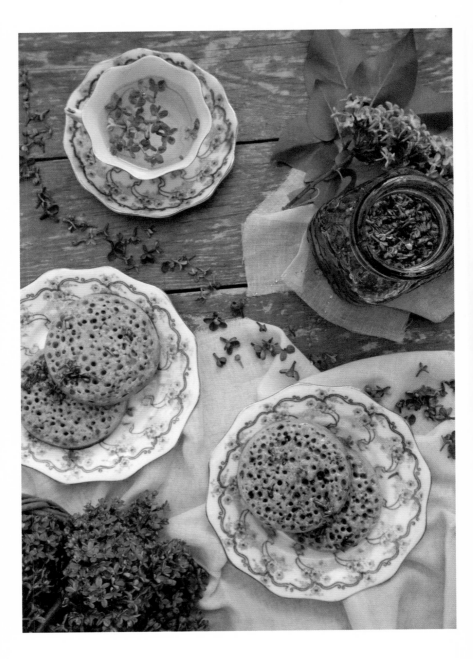

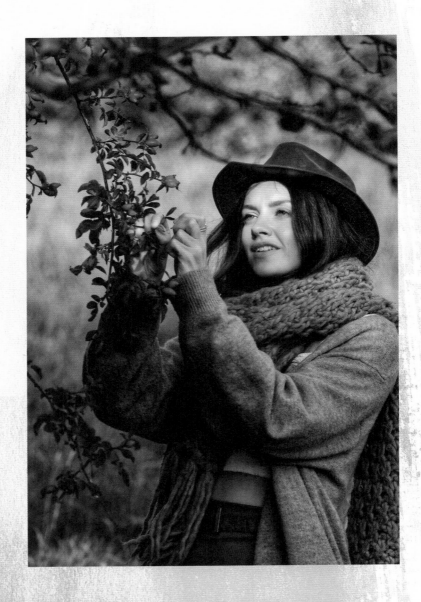

Introduction

You wander through woodland, crisp leaves crunching underfoot, blackbirds warbling in the treetops. You glance over the sun-dappled ground and see a carpet of golden brown leaves. You smell rich, damp soil, touch the rough bark of trees as you pass and breathe deeply.

After some time, you spot what looks like a cluster of bright yellow leaves and move closer to inspect them. Exhilaration and pride wash over you as you recognise some wonderful edible mushrooms. You sink your fingers into the fallen leaves, pop the golden treasures out of the earth and place them in your basket to take home. There you transform them into a delicious dish to share with your loved ones.

A connection to nature is something we all desperately need in these modern times. Social media saps our essential life force and desk jobs stunt our natural human motions and freedoms. Foraging, in my opinion, is the best way to connect, on a deep and instinctive level, with the natural world. It's not only the days spent rambling over fields and along hedgerow, the hours spent studying and appreciating how one plant differs to its neighbour and the precious moments tasting the treasures of the earth that are of value. It's also what you learn along the way – the ancient stories of the plants, their folkloric uses and their hidden meanings create a richness of experience that brings joy to the heart.

Foraging is, in some ways, the antithesis of modernity, of quick consumerism and fast food. It's about living slowly, searching for deeper meaning and enjoying the lost, the ancient, the undervalued and the wonderful.

About me

Foraging encompasses everything I love to do: spending time in the great outdoors, cooking wholesome, beautiful food, learning and sharing amazing and inspiring tales from history, anthropology and folklore.

I started foraging with my family on the South Downs when I was a kid. We used to go out on long walks, collect one of each type of mushroom we came across and take them home. There, we'd spread them out over the kitchen table and leaf through dusty old books until we got a positive identification. And that was that: I was hooked! I taught myself a lot about foraging, herbalism and wild food and learned plenty from some truly inspiring teachers – especially during my travels through Spain and Portugal, where I stayed with self-sufficient ecocommunities living in harmony with the land – until I felt confident to start sharing my knowledge.

I now run various workshops, including guided foraging walks and woodland lunches, where we walk and learn about the edible, medicinal and historical uses of the plants around us before heading back to camp to cook our foraged ingredients over a wood fire. For a long time, I was just learning, eating only the very beginner-friendly mushrooms, like giant puffballs and penny buns. It took me some months to get to know them and to be able to tell them apart from their poisonous lookalikes. And that's how it should be – foraging is all about the journey.

I hope so much that my love of foraging, sprinkled within these pages, inspires you to try it for yourself. So come with me on a journey through the woods, over the fields and back to your kitchen. Take a deep breath, reconnect with nature, discover the joy of seasonal eating and use the healing power of plants for self-care. Let the wild magic begin.

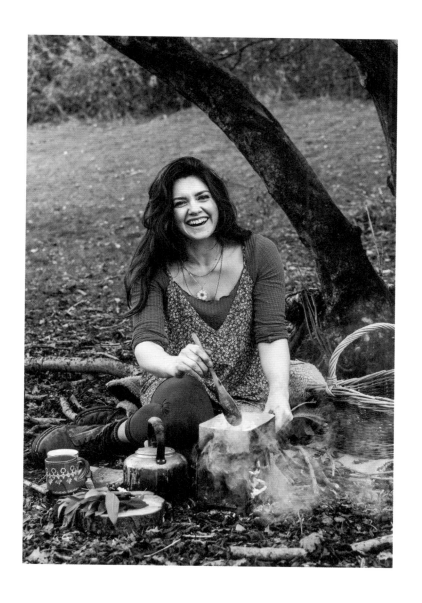

The Magic Of Foraging

The Wild Way – reconnecting with the natural world

It's easy to head to the supermarket at any time of year and fill your trolley with goodies. As you walk in you are greeted with a warm blast of air from huge, rattling air-conditioning units that ensure the shop floor is consistently tepid throughout the year. Your boots won't get muddy and strawberries are available even in winter. It's fantastically convenient but there's not much to discover in those long supermarket aisles.

It's quite the opposite when you trade your trolley for a foraging basket. Those shelves stacked with plastic packets are now tall trees, a fresh breeze running through them with a comforting rustle. Sometimes they're vibrant with a thousand green leaves, sometimes those leaves are in tones of golden brown, red and purple as they fall to cover the forest floor. Sometimes they are bare and stark, luminescent with the touch of frost. No matter how they are dressed, they are always there for you and always have some wisdom to impart.

While foraging is essentially about harvesting from nature, I want to let you in on a secret … it's not all about the harvest. In fact, sometimes I don't take anything, yet return home just as happy. Almost every time I post a picture of my latest foraged goods, people ask me where I found them. It would be easy to tell them, of course, but to inform the fledgling forager of the exact location of the wild ingredients would be to deprive them of the magical and valuable journey of learning to forage, robbing them of a thousand squishy footprints through the mud, hundreds of moments filled with birdsong and sun glare,

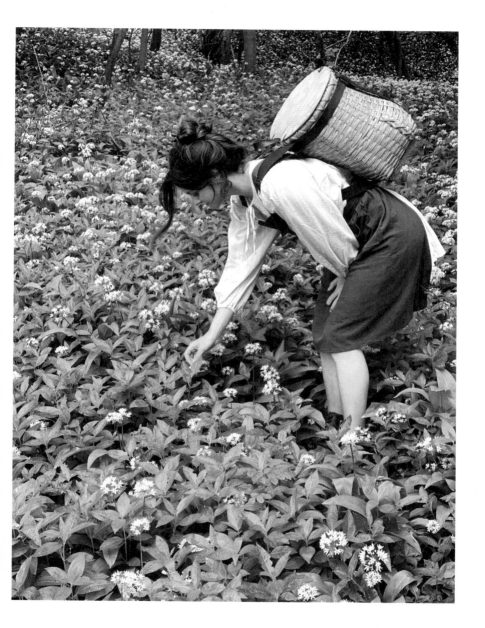

tens of frustrating 'unsuccessful' hunts and that one truly spectacular moment when they found what they were looking for, with their own intuition and newfound foraging prowess.

Every foraging session is the start of an adventure. As your trusty foraging guide, *Wild Magic* will take you into little antique shops to find your perfect basket and over the fields and meadows to find long-lost ingredients. It will take you back in time to understand the secret power of the plants around us, and the stories and ancient uses of our wildflowers, fruits, herbs and vegetables.

The nature cure – the connection between nature and mental health

The benefits of nature have been well documented – there are plenty of studies that show that time spent in nature has a positive effect on physical and mental health. For instance, in Japan, forest bathing, or *shinrin-yoku*, is often prescribed by doctors for patients suffering from stress, overwhelm and depression. Patients are encouraged to spend time in nature, using their senses to interact with the natural environment mindfully. It's no wonder that the natural world has such a huge benefit on mental health. If we condensed the whole of human history into one day, we only stopped foraging around an hour and 20 minutes ago. That's a lot of time spent foraging and living our lives so closely intertwined with nature. In that time, our bodies evolved to become natural foragers – roaming the land with our tribe to gather and harvest wild foods is our natural state.

That's why I think foraging brings such a deep joy: because, unlike sitting at a desk all day, we're letting our body do something that is so natural to us. It feels like coming home.

Ancient magic

No matter who you are, no matter what your heritage, your ancestors were foragers and this is something that connects us. I often feel like I'm walking in the footsteps of my ancestors, collecting herbs and berries and concocting them into potions and broths at home. I try to think about how they would have used the plants around us and love looking into the ancient magic and medicinal uses. I imagine that the wise women who came before me crushed the same spices, brewed the same herbs and whispered and sung their words while stirring their stews like I do.

Many wild plants are steeped in ancient folklore too and discovering these age-old stories is one of my favourite things to do. They may have once been the disguise of a Greek goddess as she tried to evade the advances an interested suitor, or perhaps a token of bad luck, which when brought inside was thought to cause death and misery. We'll be exploring some of these wonderful folk tales along with the edible uses of wild plants.

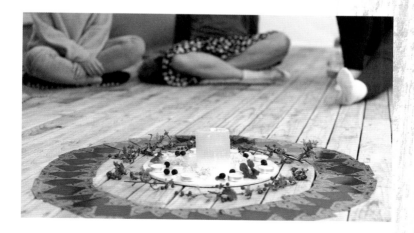

The healing powers of plants

Foraged food = fresh food

Plants picked and eaten the same day are highly nutritious. For instance, some studies show that vegetables can lose 15–55 per cent of their vitamin C content within a week, while spinach can even lose 90 per cent of its vitamin C content just 24 hours after being harvested. Foraging is a great way to make sure you're eating freshly picked foods.

Wild spaces = nutrient-rich soil

Modern agricultural methods have also stripped much of the soil of its nutrients, which leads to less nutrient-rich foods. A landmark US study on the topic used nutritional data from both 1950 and 1999 for 43 different vegetables and fruits, finding 'reliable declines' in the amount of protein, calcium, phosphorus, iron, riboflavin (vitamin B2) and vitamin C over the past half century. Our wild spaces are generally undisturbed, meaning the soil is packed with nutrients which carry through to the wild plants.

A varied diet

For their book *Ikigai: The Japanese Secret to a Long and Happy Life*, Francesc Miralles and Héctor García studied the ways of the people living in Okinawa, a town which boasts the record for being home to the longest-living people. They found that the local people ate a huge variety of foods (a lot of them being freshly picked from vegetable gardens) in comparison to typical Western diets and they believed this was a contributing factor to their overall health.

Foraging gives you access to not only a huge number of ingredients, but ingredients that are very different from the usual suspects that end up in supermarket trolleys week after week.

Plant medicine

Medicinal plants have been used in traditional medicine for thousands of years and our ancestors certainly knew the benefits of certain plants to heal. We now live in an era of manufactured medicines, but many of the drugs that are considered key today are derived from plants, from morphine and codeine to quinine. Worldwide, between 50,000 and 80,000 flowering plants are used medicinally, and in the United States, of the top 150 prescription drugs, at least 118 are based on natural sources. However, while there is no doubt that these manufactured drugs have had many benefits, many of us are drawn to the medicinal plants that started it all, looking at ways that herbal remedies can boost our physical and mental wellbeing.

When we look at these factors together, it's clear that wild plants can offer us incredible healing powers. I hope you will start to look at those little patches of weeds a bit differently!

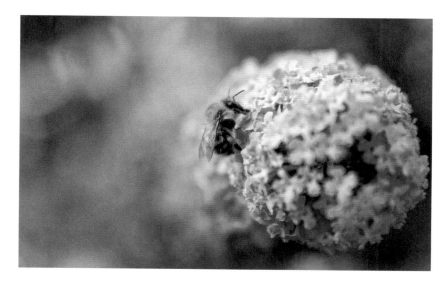

How to Forage Responsibly

Sustainability

I firmly believe that there is no group of people more likely to want to protect and nurture their wild spaces than the people who harvest their food from it. Foraging can be done sustainably, but the onus of sustainable foraging is one of upmost importance, that we all must take a responsibility for.

The more you forage, the more you will form a deep connection with the natural world, and begin to understand the natural cycles and balance of all things. But when we're just beginning our foraging journeys, we could cause harm without knowing we've even done so. Here are some important rules to follow to make sure you are foraging sustainably:

1. Take time to learn about the specific plant or mushroom you're interested in before you start to harvest them. Make sure they are common in your area, and research how they spread, so you can leave plenty of their reproductive parts or help distribute them! For example, mushrooms should only be picked at maturity, to give them a chance to spread their spores and are always best gathered in wicker baskets, so we can help them spread their spores as we walk through the woods.
2. Only ever harvest what you need from abundant areas (if there's only a few of something, don't take any). When you're foraging, be careful not to overharvest one area. Pick a little and move on, leaving plenty for wildlife.

3. Let nature show you what she has enough of with a display of abundance. There's no use heading out with a set-in-stone idea of what you want to forage and cook, because it might lead to overharvesting something that there simply isn't enough of. It's much better to see what there's a lot of, and then work out what you can make with that!
4. Be respectful of the plants and animals around you when you harvest. It's fine to pick from an abundant bramble bush, but not when you trample over wildflowers to get there! Be aware that animals use large hedges as walkways, so don't take big areas back completely, just snip a little of the top and sides – like you're giving that hedgerow a haircut!
5. Give back! There are so many ways to give back to nature: you could support a local wildlife charity, you could spread native bee-friendly wildflower seeds in your local hedgerows or you could grow flowers in your garden throughout the summer.

Communing with plants

We might think of plants as being unconscious resources, but they are so much more than that. Like all living things, plants have their own frequencies and can even sense their surroundings, whether it's a drop of rain or a tap of a finger on a leaf.

Whether you consider them conscious entities or not, I encourage you to take a moment to commune with the plants before harvesting anything. This can be as simple as taking a moment to quietly focus on the plant, asking if you can take some of what it has to offer.

Adding this meditative element to your foraging practice will help you to forage more consciously and deepen your connection to nature.

The law

The laws around foraging are notoriously vague and will differ from country to country. Having a good understanding of the laws that allow you to forage will make you feel confident when you're out harvesting your wild foods.

In the UK, section 4 of the Property and Theft Act states that: 'A person who picks mushrooms growing wild on any land, or who picks flowers, fruit or foliage from a plant growing wild on any land, does not (although not in possession of the land) steal what he picks, unless he does it for reward or for sale or other commercial purpose.'

This law is more commonly known as the law of the four Fs and allows us to forage for fruits, flowers, fungi and foliage, providing they are not protected plants, they are for personal use and they are growing wild. This law, however, does not trump the trespassing law and if you are on private land and are asked to leave, you must do so. It also does not trump any bylaws that the local council or conservation groups may have put in place (i.e. do not pick or remove any flora). These bylaws will be displayed on posters in the areas they apply to.

You should also be aware that it is illegal to uproot any plant without permission from the landowner. In the UK, public footpaths and council-owned land are good places to start.

In the US, foraging laws differ from state to state. Some allow foraging on any public land and others prohibit the practice in city parks. When it comes to national parks, 46 out of the 56 parks allow some foraging (usually with some limitations as to what you can forage in place), while 14 parks have banned it entirely. So if you're planning a hike to forage some food, make sure you plan which park you go to accordingly!

In the majority of Europe, including France and Germany, there is much more freedom when it comes to foraging. In France you can forage on any public land so long as there are no local bylaws in place. In Germany you're not permitted to forage in protected parks but can forage in public areas.

Please remember that it's your responsibility to check on your local foraging laws before you head off to fill your basket.

Safety

I cannot emphasise enough how important it is that you are 100 per cent certain about the identity of any plant that you will cook, serve and eat. For some plants this will be easy, as almost everyone knows what a nettle or a blackberry looks like. For other plants, this will take a little more time, research and practice.

It's also important to be respectful and mindful when harvesting wild plants. Most cases of wild food poisoning in the UK come from 'clumsy' foraging. Here are some useful tips to help you protect yourself:

1. Avoid grabbing big handfuls of your chosen ingredient as you could have a little piece of deadly hemlock caught up in your harvest. Go slowly and carefully check everything you pick.
2. Make sure you pick from areas that haven't been sprayed with pesticides and away from busy roads.
3. When you're trying out a new wild ingredient, especially mushrooms, just have a little to start with in case you have an intolerance you're not aware of. If your body is happy then that's great!
4. When foraging for mushrooms, as well as being sure you've identified them correctly (see page 24), make sure you are picking a mushroom in the prime of its life. Occasionally I hear from people who have got sick after eating perfectly 'edible' mushrooms. However, when they sent me the photo of the mushroom they ate, it was well past its prime, losing colour and almost rotting on the tree.

Friendly Foraging:
The Four Rules

Rule 1
Never eat anything unless you're 100 per cent sure you have correctly identified an edible plant.

Rule 2
Only ever harvest small amounts from areas of abundance. If there's only a little of something, don't take any.

Rule 3
Harvest carefully; don't grab big handfuls as poisonous weeds may get entangled.

Rule 4
Be mindful and respectful of the plants, animals and people around you.

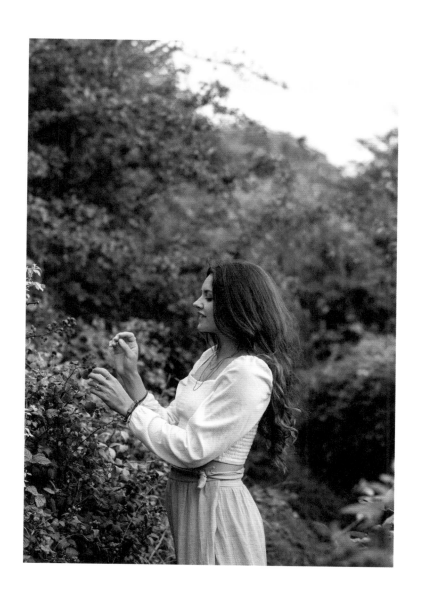

How to ID a new plant

I know that when you start your foraging journey, things can seem a little daunting. Looking over meadows seems more like observing a sea of green, rather than individual plants you might one day know the names of. But I promise you, with time and patience, you'll recognise each little herb like an old friend.

To start identifying new plants, you'll need to use all the resources available to you, such as plant ID apps, Facebook groups and field guides. Start with just one herb, berry or mushroom that you feel drawn to. Take photos or pick a small sample of your chosen wild thing and study it closely.

Upload your photos to your plant ID app to give you the first clue as to what you might have. (Note: I do NOT recommend plant ID apps for foraging purposes, but they are great at giving you a place to start.) Then look through your field guides to see if you agree with the app's ID. You can also post your photos to Facebook ID groups to get help from other members (there are hundreds of foraging groups on Facebook, it's best to find one based in your area so the other members are more likely to know what you have).

Using all of these clues, you'll be able to reach a place of confidence in your identification of your chosen plant. With time, you'll be so confident in your identification skills, you'll be eating your edible finds. Congratulations!

When I started my foraging journey, I really loved scrapbooking, so I would draw the plant and press samples to stick in my journal. Once I had identified it, I would write what I had, it's unique characteristics, and any little titbits of folklore I could find on it too.

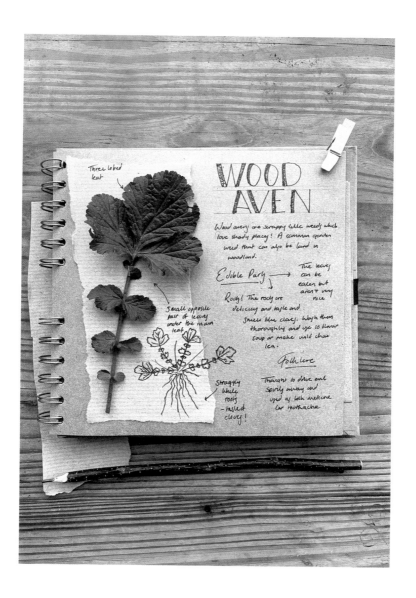

Three lobed leaf

WOOD AVEN

Wood aveny are scrappy little weedy which love shady placey! A common garden weed that can also be found in woodland.

Edible Party → The leaves can be eaten but aren't very nice

Rooty! The rooty are delicious and taple and smell like clovey. Waph them thoroughly and use to flavour soup or make wild chai tea.

Small opposite pair of leaves under the main leaf

Straggly white roots – tasted clovey!

Folklore

Thought to drive evil spirity away and used as folk medicine for toothache

How to ID a new mushroom

I hear so many people describing the journey to foraging and eating their first wild mushroom as 'scary', but it really shouldn't be this way. Remember, there is absolutely no rush to eat anything. Half the journey is in learning about the plant, or in this case the mushroom, and it's such an enjoyable journey.

When I first started looking into foraging mushrooms I was completely nonplussed after reading sentences like 'This mushroom has a fluffy skirt' and 'This mushroom has a white volva'. (Yes, really!) So, first let's look at the structure of a mushroom and what the different parts are called so these sentences make a little more sense.

The anatomy of a mushroom

On the opposite page you'll see a diagram of a mushroom and its different features, note that not all mushrooms will have all of these features. For example, sometimes a mushroom might be listed as having a 'simple stipe' which means it has no volva, and no skirt. It's the combination of features a mushroom does, or doesn't have, along with where it grows, its colour and its texture that makes it unique and identifiable.

Spore Printing

Spore printing is a great way to make sure you have correctly identified your mushroom. Mushrooms drop spores, which are like microscopic seeds, from their gills, pores or teeth. These spores differ in colour from mushroom to mushroom, from white to black and in shades of red, lilacs and even greens. They give us a final clue so we can establish if we have a correct ID. This isn't always necessary, but can be very helpful if the mushroom you're looking for has toxic lookalikes. You might have checked all the features of the mushroom and feel fairly confident, but need that one final check. A spore print is that check!

How to take a spore print:

1. Take the mushroom you are looking to identify and cut away the stipe so you have only the cap.
2. Place it on a sheet of paper. If you know the colour of the spore you are looking for, use a paper that will highlight that colour, for example black paper for white spores. If you're unsure, place the cap so it's sitting on half a piece of white and half a piece of black paper.
3. Place a bowl, cup or glass over the cap so it doesn't dry out and leave it for 12–24 hours.

The anatomy of a mushroom

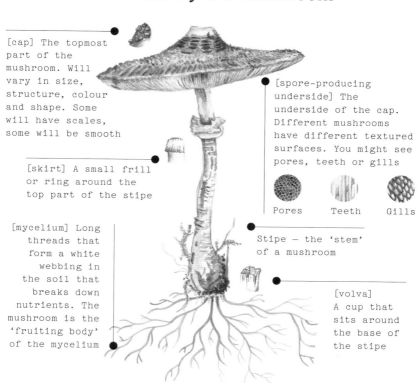

[cap] The topmost part of the mushroom. Will vary in size, structure, colour and shape. Some will have scales, some will be smooth

[spore-producing underside] The underside of the cap. Different mushrooms have different textured surfaces. You might see pores, teeth or gills

Pores   Teeth   Gills

[skirt] A small frill or ring around the top part of the stipe

[mycelium] Long threads that form a white webbing in the soil that breaks down nutrients. The mushroom is the 'fruiting body' of the mycelium

Stipe — the 'stem' of a mushroom

[volva] A cup that sits around the base of the stipe

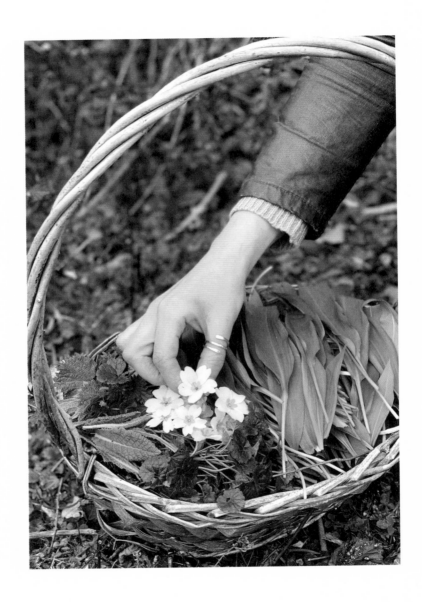

Foraging Equipment

The great thing about foraging is you really don't need any kit to get started. It can be as simple as walking to your local hedgerow or overgrown alleyway, equipped with a Tupperware box to collect blackberries. If you're anything like me though, the more into foraging you get, the more appealing those superfluous, yet handy items will become. As I have an inkling some of you will be drawn to them too, here's some information on all of these tools, plus a few extras that might take your fancy.

Baskets

Baskets are fantastic things. They come in all shapes and sizes and I'm sure you'll end up with a collection and a favourite. If you're buying new, I highly recommend looking out for a local basket maker. They should be easy to find via a quick internet search, or you can find them at your nearest village or craft fair – or support an independent maker or seller via Instagram, Depop, eBay, Etsy or even Gumtree. You can also find baskets easily in charity shops, at flea markets and car-boot sales.

Muslin foraging bags

Muslin foraging bags definitely aren't a necessity, but they're a great way to keep your foraging basket organised. Without them, you'll be spending a long time organising messy heaps of herbs and wildflowers when you get home after a forage. Of course, you could also use glass jars or smaller baskets if you'd prefer.

Knives

Knives are fantastic for harvesting wild herbs while minimising the risk of uprooting the plant. Some come with little brushes on the end; these are for brushing dirt off mushrooms, which don't like to be washed.

In the UK you are not allowed to carry a knife in public without a 'valid reason', unless it has a folding blade that is less that 8cm (3in) long, so I would always recommend a small, folding knife. Make sure you are aware of the law on carrying knives wherever you live.

Gloves

Gloves are great for protecting your hands from getting too dry and rough and gardening gloves are a good option; however, if you're picking nettles, I must warn you the sting goes right through! For picking stingers I recommend incredibly embarrassing but wonderfully effective … washing-up gloves!

Gardening trowel and secateurs

Secateurs and a small trowel will come in handy for snipping sturdy stems – you probably already have a pair of secateurs if you garden from time to time.

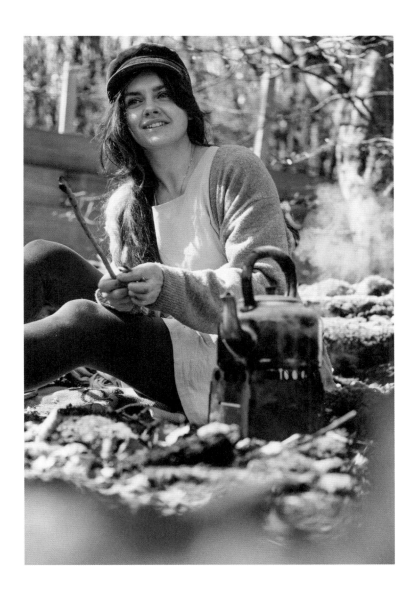

A NOTE ON THE RECIPES

Most of the recipes found in this book can be made plant-based with simple swaps. I personally use dairy-free alternatives to milk, butter and cheese in my own recipes, usually made from nuts, but haven't felt the need to list each ingredient as 'plant-based cheese' and so on. Although I use local, organic eggs, you can substitute the egg with a chia or flax egg, or aquafaba (the water from a tin of chickpeas) depending on your preference.

To make 1 plant-based 'egg', combine 1 tablespoon of ground flaxseed (or chia seed) and 3 tablespoons of water. Allow to sit for 10 minutes until you have a gloopy gel. Use this as you would an egg.

Most of my recipes include one wild ingredient per recipe; I like keeping my recipes simple like this because it makes foraging more accessible and showcases the wild product on hand.

I encourage you to get creative with these recipes, switching out or adding in other wild ingredients.

Working with wild ingredients is not the same as working with shop-bought ingredients. In supermarkets, fruits and vegetables are pretty much the same across the board, but the same can not be said for wild foods. There are also many subspecies of plants within one species – for example, there are many different varieties of crab apple! Remember to taste your ingredients as you go, picking only the tastiest; you may need to adjust the sugar and acid levels accordingly in these recipes.

You'll also need to learn to pick wild foods in their prime. For example, hawthorns are ready when they're dark red and easily squashed between finger and thumb. Trying to make hawthorn ketchup with underripe hawthorns won't result in a very nice dish!

A NOTE ON THE PLANTS

Not all of the plants in this book are considered 'wild'; lavender and magnolia, for example, are popular garden plants which we don't often find in our wild spaces. However, I have decided that these not-so-wild plants deserve a space among the rest. Think of them as 'gateway plants' if you will. Growing up in fairly urban areas, when I first started foraging it took me a while to build up the courage to pick plants from the wild. They seemed so unknown and unattainable. Starting your foraging journey with plants that you might find in the garden is a brilliant way to begin. You'll experience that joy of spending time outdoors, harvesting plants and making something from scratch! You can go on and build up your foraging prowess from there.

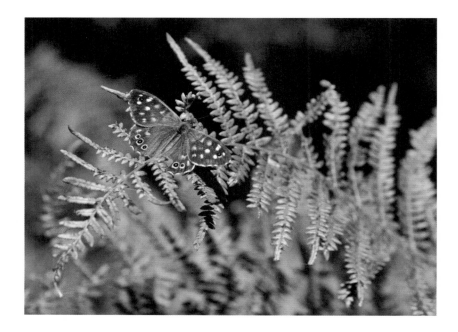

Spring

Over the meadows and in the woodlands, where once there was only bare branches and exposed earth, life begins to stir. The smallest of buds appear on the trees and vibrant green shoots break their way through soil and snow. This new life elicits a hushed wonder, as if anything louder or coarser could scare it away. Wrens and great tits who have seen out the winter warble their anticipation at the season yet to come.

Spring is slow at first, a whisper that you can hear in the trees. It happens out of sight, under the earth and within strong trunks. Plants that have been slumbering are awakening and their bright, vibrant energy surges upwards once more, until life floods the land and the world is a cottage garden once more.

Hedgerow plants rise up and burst open in celebration. Tall and merry stands of cow parsley offer lacy clouds of flowers as decoration for the event. Woodland banks are draped in colour. Yellow primroses and lilac bluebells bloom with joy. Tiny wild violets, dropped like gems on the earth, bob their heads on graceful swan-like necks, peeking through carpets of wild garlic.

Spring is a time to celebrate the return of life and immerse yourself in the jubilant festivities of nature.

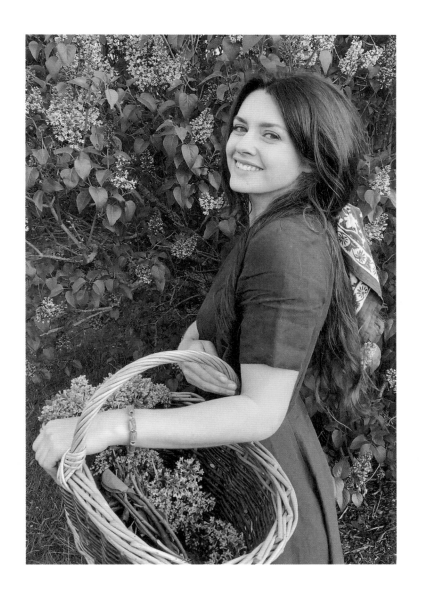

Foraging in Spring

Spring is a time of plenty, so of course there's plenty of foraging to be done! I rarely buy a bag of salad during this bountiful season and every dish is garnished with a wildflower or two. The vibrancy and freshness of nature delight me while I forage, linger like a happy dream while I cook and taste like sunshine as I eat. I love to cook and eat outside during the spring, to be as close as possible to the plants that nourish me so deeply. Whether it's wild herb flatbreads on the griddle, hot potato salad with wild garlic on the campfire or simply a fresh handful of wild greens to pop into my sandwich, it's a perfect way to immerse yourself in nature and celebrate the emergence of spring.

Fresh spring greens

One of my favourite springtime sights is a grassy bank covered in wild edible greens. It is so rewarding to potter through the various sprouts, picking sprigs here and there until you have a basket filled with nutritious, tasty greens! From nettles to sticky weed, they all offer different flavours and textures and it's such a pleasure to get to know them all as ingredients.

Almost all of the spring greens I mention on page 38 can be used interchangeably in a range of recipes, including pesto, green juice, sautéed greens, fresh salads, green soups, stews and curries. Remember to learn about each green individually, as some will need to be cooked before using, some will be more bitter than others and some you'll want to use more as a herb for flavouring, whereas others can be served by the bowlful like a salad leaf.

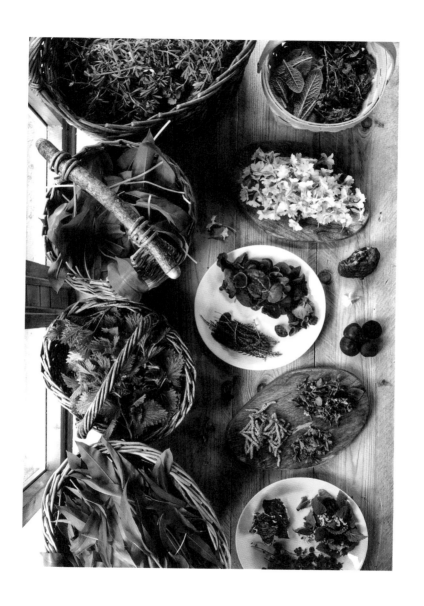

Many wild greens will be much more flavoursome than your average salad leaf and will offer a wide range of vitamins and nutrients. When harvesting spring greens, pick only the freshest sprigs and leave plenty behind, so the plant can continue to flourish.

Here is a list of my favourite spring greens:

Wild garlic
Cleavers
Nettles
Chickweed
Ground ivy
Ground elder
Primrose leaves
Few-flowered leek
Three-cornered leek

Jack-by-the-hedge
Cow parsley
Sea beet
Hogweed
Mallow
Sorrel
Common vetch
Dandelion
Lamb's quarters

Flowers

There is an ancient Chinese proverb that says, 'If you have two loaves, sell one and buy a lily'. It attests to the idea that we need food to sustain the body, but we also need beauty to sustain the soul. So it must be true that eating flowers feeds both the body and the soul – I certainly think so anyway!

Flowers are one of my favourite things to collect in spring, whether to cook with or use for rituals. They bring a delicate beauty to any dish, whether used as a garnish on a salad, or infused in a syrup or gin to impart their elegant flavours. A handful of fresh flowers sprinkled on top of a warm bath on a spring evening is the perfect way to bring some wild charm to your bathing routine.

It's always best to harvest flowers in the morning of a sunny day, while the dew is still upon them and before their pollen has been swept away by the wind, or collected by pollinators.

Remember that flowers are very important to our pollinators and are the reproductive part of the plant, so we should only take a few flowers here and there when we see a huge abundance of them. To harvest flowers in a sustainable way, only pick around one flower for every twenty that you see.

I like to balance out what I take from the wild by planting more flowers in my garden! You can buy specific native pollinator-friendly flowers which ensures you're giving back in the right way. You can also spread some native wildflower seed in your local meadows – find out how to make your own wild seed bombs on page 103!

The language of flowers

Foraging for flowers is so much more than what we gain or create from them. It's what we learn as we study them too. Flowers have always been adored and used in so many disciplines, whether art, literature, medicine, cosmetics, magical and religious symbolism or fashion.

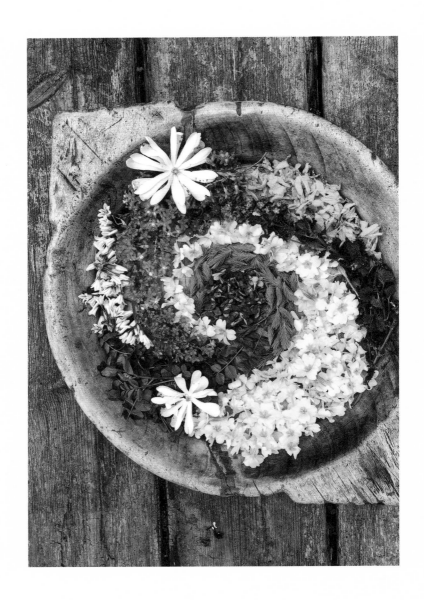

One of my favourite ways that flowers have been used, is through the language of the flowers. Meaning has been attributed to flowers for thousands of years but it was the Victorians who popularised the tradition of sending posies of flowers, in which each flower had its own meaning, thereby including a message or a riddle. By studying which flowers were in the posy and the meaning of those flowers one could unpick the riddle. Here are some of my favourites:

PRIMROSE	youthfulness or young love
LAVENDER	purity, devotion and caution
DOG ROSE	simplicity
RED ROSE	deep and passionate love
PINK ROSE	warm, sibling-like affection
YELLOW ROSE	jealousy and infidelity
VIOLET	innocence and shyness
LILAC	flirtatious, playful romantic interest

The Victorian obsession with flowers drew from many other cultures; for example the yellow rose seems to have the same meaning in the Islamic world. One legend describes how the Prophet Mohammed, suspecting his wife of adultery, tosses a bouquet of red roses into a pool and they turn yellow, confirming her guilt.

Whenever I meet a new flower, I always spend some time learning about what it has meant to other people and other cultures. Somehow it adds a layer of complexity and magic to my floral dishes!

Wild Garlic

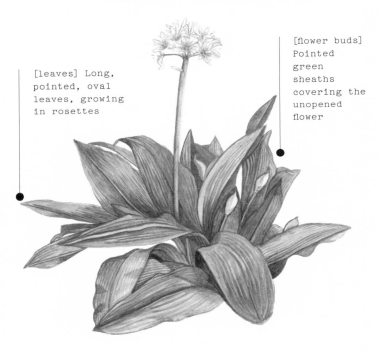

[leaves] Long, pointed, oval leaves, growing in rosettes

[flower buds] Pointed green sheaths covering the unopened flower

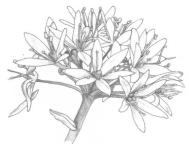

[flower] White star-shaped flowers which open in the summer

Foraging notes

Wild garlic is a firm favourite with so many foragers and chefs and it's really no wonder. It grows so abundantly, usually covering vast areas, and has the most wonderful fresh, garlicky flavour that is released when crushed. So, if you're wandering through the woods and smell garlic, this might be the tasty culprit.

Wild garlic loves damp, shady environments and can often be found on the outskirts of woodland or lining streams. The leaves start popping up in early spring, in late spring the unopened buds appear and then burst open into flowers – by summer it's mostly gone.

Once wild garlic leaves are fully grown, there's really nothing you can get them confused with, especially if you make an effort to smell each one before it goes in the basket. There are no toxic members of the allium (onion/garlic) family, so if it smells garlicky, you're safe. The closest toxic lookalike is a plant called lily of the valley, which has similar shaped leaves, but they don't smell of garlic.

When wild garlic leaves are very small, they could be confused with the leaves of young lords and ladies (*Arum maculatum*) plants; these are toxic so make sure they don't make their way into your basket! Again, they don't smell of garlic, but they do like to grow in similar environments to wild garlic. This should serve as a reminder to forage mindfully and carefully. Harvest leaf by leaf, don't grab big handfuls.

So you can keep coming back for more, only harvest between three and five nice big leaves from each wild garlic plant and a few buds or flowers from each. You can also use the unopened flower buds and flowers, but remember they are the reproductive part of the plant so leave plenty behind.

Wild garlic recipes

Don't bother digging up wild garlic bulbs, it's the leaves, buds and flowers that are the stars of the show. They can be eaten fresh, stirred into salads, pickled, puréed or used in a sauce or marinade. There's not much you can't do with them! Try the following recipes, replace them with the other wild greens in this book, and if you'd like even more options, try pickling the unopened wild garlic buds by following the recipe for pickled magnolia petals on page 55.

Plant lore, folk medicine & magic

Wild garlic makes a few appearances in Irish folklore. Remains of wild garlic cloves have been found in ancient thatch roofing and were thought to be placed there to protect the house from evil spirits and mischievous fairies. It's also known as 'bears' garlic' as it was thought to be the favourite food of brown bears coming out of hibernation. In Celtic culture, wild garlic was known as 'The Healing Herb' and, like regular garlic, it is thought to help lower blood cholesterol and has antibacterial and antifungal properties.

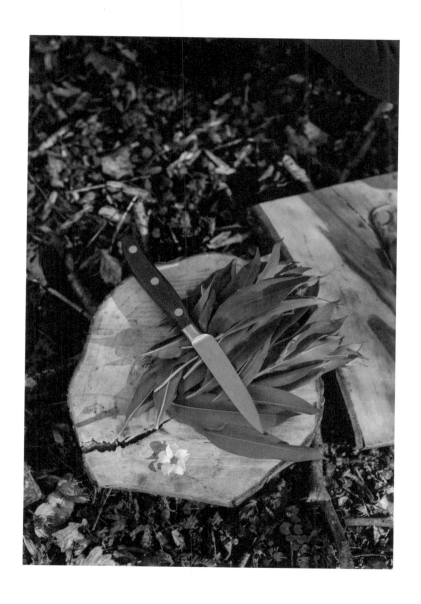

Wild garlic butter

Pickles, pestos, sauerkrauts and kimchis are fantastic options for preserving your wild garlic, but they also change the flavour quite a bit. If it's the middle of winter, and you want the pure, unadulterated taste of wild garlic, then wild garlic butter is the one for you. It keeps in the fridge for at least a few months and it freezes for up to a year. Just take it out of the freezer to defrost a couple of hours before you're ready to use it.

I've tried this recipe with dairy and non-dairy butter (not margarine) and it works wonderfully with both. Simply spread it on toast or wild garlic muffins (see opposite), cook with it, or let a generous sliver melt over your favourite pasta dish – my favourite is on top of wild mushroom ravioli (see page 215).

MAKES 225G (8OZ)

225g (8oz) block of butter, softened
Handful of wild garlic leaves, chopped (see Note)
Salt and freshly ground black pepper

1. Make sure you remove your butter from the fridge a few hours before you make this so it is soft enough to blend. Add the butter to a bowl and blend in a handful or two of wild garlic, depending on how garlicky you want it! Season with salt and pepper.
2. Once blended, plop it on to a square of parchment paper and form into a sausage shape in the middle of the square.
3. Fold the paper over the sausage and tuck it in. Roll the paper fairly tightly around the butter and then twist both ends like you're making a wrapped sweet.
4. Pop it into the fridge and leave to chill for a few hours. Voila! A beautiful roll of wild garlic butter.

NOTE
I like to shred my wild garlic with a knife and mix it in by hand, to retain some of the wild garlic texture. When you do it like this it creates a beautiful marbled pattern in the butter. You can also blend it in a food processor and then mix it in, creating a super-vibrant green butter.

Wild garlic muffins

Wild garlic muffins have a soft, buttery texture, the pungent taste of garlic and smooth rich taste of Cheddar cheese. The simple ritual of creating them always makes me happy.

Whenever I'm in the mood to bake it's often a toss-up between scones and muffins; invariably muffins win. Here's my go-to recipe for six delicious wild garlic muffins.

MAKES 6

1 medium egg, beaten
50ml (2fl oz) melted butter or vegetable oil, plus extra for greasing
125ml (½ cup) milk
125g (1 cup) self-raising flour
½ tsp baking powder
100g (3½oz) grated Cheddar
Handful of chopped wild garlic
Sea salt and freshly ground black pepper

1. Preheat the oven to 200°C/400°F/gas 6 and lightly grease the insides of a six-hole muffin tin with oil.
2. Add the beaten egg, melted butter or oil and milk to a jug and stir together. In a separate bowl, mix together all the remaining ingredients.
3. Pour the wet ingredients into the bowl and stir together to make a smooth batter, then spoon evenly into the muffin tin.
4. Bake for about 25 minutes until the tops are golden brown.
5. This recipe would also work with lots of other flavoursome wild greens – try it with three-cornered leek, jack-by-the-hedge, ground ivy or nettles (but do steam your nettles for a few minutes before using in this recipe).

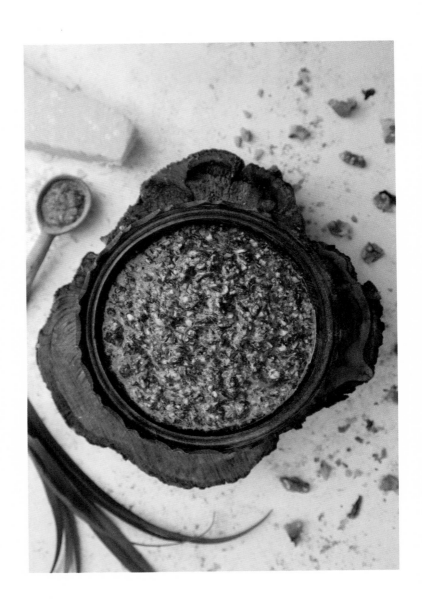

Wild garlic pesto

This is my go-to recipe for any abundant green, whether it be three-cornered leek, wild garlic, or even lightly steamed nettles. There are so many recipes out there for wild greens pesto, but it is an essential and can be used in so many ways, from pasta dishes to salad dressings to a dip for fresh veggies, so it deserves a place here.

There are two options here: you can either make this in a food processor or chop everything finely by hand.

MAKES ROUGHLY 1 JAR

2 large bunches of wild garlic leaves
60g (2½oz) pine nuts, toasted
Juice of 1 lemon
60g (2½oz) Parmesan cheese, grated
150ml (5fl oz) good-quality olive oil

1. If you are using a food processor, roughly chop the wild garlic leaves first so that they don't clog the blades. Add to the food processor along with the pine nuts, lemon juice and grated Parmesan. Blitz until you have a smoothish paste, then gradually pour in the oil and blitz again. This will give you a super-fine, almost creamy pesto which is great for coating pasta.

2. Alternatively, chop the wild garlic leaves and pine nuts finely by hand, then transfer to a bowl and whisk in the lemon juice, Parmesan and oil. This will give you a chunkier pesto.

3. Wild garlic pesto will last for up to a week in the fridge and up to 6 months in the freezer.

Magnolia

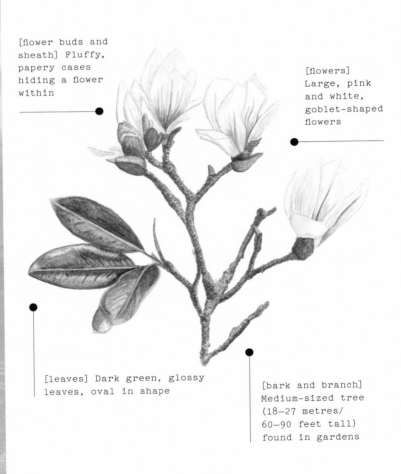

[flower buds and sheath] Fluffy, papery cases hiding a flower within

[flowers] Large, pink and white, goblet-shaped flowers

[leaves] Dark green, glossy leaves, oval in shape

[bark and branch] Medium-sized tree (18—27 metres/ 60—90 feet tall) found in gardens

Foraging notes

Magnolias are huge, beautiful trees native to China. They're a common garden plant here in the UK, so aren't really 'wild', but it's important to focus on what's abundant, not what's native! Magnolias have been a food source in China for centuries and now that they're here, we may as well make the most of them.

There are many varieties of magnolia and none are known to have any toxicity. It's best to stick with the varieties that have been tested and certified edible, so here we'll focus on one of the most common: *Magnolia* x *soulangeana*. However, if you google 'List of edible magnolia flowers' you will find a full list of tested varieties.

Magnolias vary in flavour across not only species but individual trees too. You'll find some have a spicy, gingery kick, while some have flavours similar to cardamom and some have hints of vanilla. Magnolia petals are edible raw so the best way to make sure you're working with one you like is to have a nibble before you start harvesting.

Magnolias are ready to harvest when the flower buds have begun to burst open. The best way to pick magnolias to eat is to simply pick off the petals, leaving the stamen, so the insects can continue to benefit from their pollen. Whole buds can be picked but the furry brown sheath should be removed.

Remember to always ask permission from the landowner when you're picking magnolias. I'm often knocking on neighbours' doors and asking if they wouldn't mind me picking a few magnolias. They're bound to say yes if you let them know they're edible and offer a jar of pickled magnolia in return!

Magnolia recipes

All parts of the magnolia flower can be eaten both raw and cooked, once the furry sheath is removed. The petals can be shredded and added to a salad, which adds a beautiful pop of colour and a hit of flavour (they can be quite strong though so be careful that they don't overpower the other flavours).

The flower petals can also be dried and made into a delicate floral tea; dried petals can also be powdered and used as a flavouring, lending ginger/cardamom notes to any dish or dessert.

Plant lore, folk medicine & magic

Fossils have revealed that magnolia plants existed at least 20 million years ago. Magnolia flowers are so big because they evolved before lots of smaller pollinators, like the bee; because of this the magnolia had to grow to match larger pollinators that were around at the time, like moths and beetles.

In ancient Chinese medicine, magnolia bark, taken as an infusion, was used as a cure for insomnia, anxiety and depression, while the flower bud was used for clearing sinus congestion and relieving sinus headaches. The flowers were thought to represent dignity and nobility.

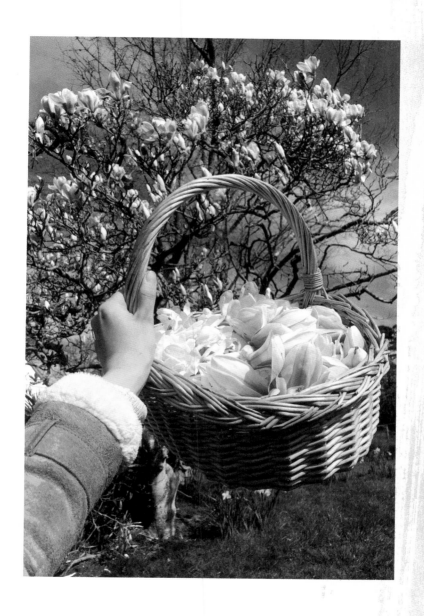

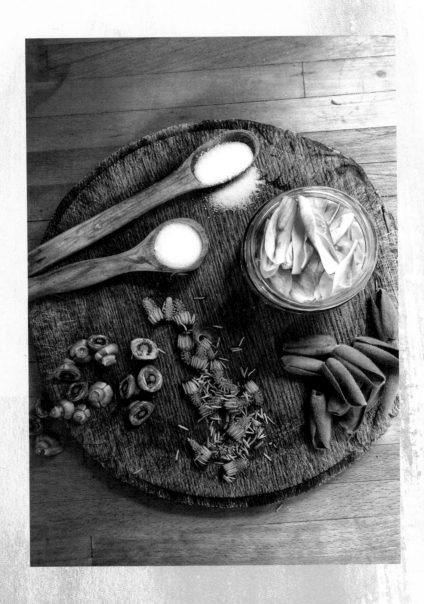

Pickled magnolia

Pickled magnolia petals taste gorgeous! You know the little packets of pickled ginger you get in sushi packs? They taste so similar to that, but with extra cardamomy, floral tones. What's more, they're so easy to make. It makes for a pickle that goes wonderfully with sushi.

I've found the best way to pack the jars is in a rose shape, that way the petals don't float to the top of the jar, but stay underneath the vinegar line! If they're above the line, they won't stay a nice pink colour.

MAKES 1 SMALL JAR

350ml (12fl oz) white wine vinegar
1 tbsp white sugar
1 tbsp salt
Approx. 20 magnolia buds or flowers (young petals with no browning or damage)

1. Sterilise a small jar – I use one that holds about 400ml (14fl oz) of liquid.
2. Pour the vinegar into a small saucepan, add the sugar and salt and place over a very low heat, stirring until the sugar and salt have dissolved. Turn off the heat and leave to cool completely.
3. Prepare your magnolia buds by removing the tough, hairy sheath surrounding the bottom of the flower. Then chop the base of the flower, which holds the petals together, and separate out the petals. You'll find a small, pineapple shape in the middle, which I tend to leave out, but you could pickle it too if you wanted.
4. Pack the jar full of magnolia petals and pour over pickling solution. If you have a pickling weight, place it on top of the petals. (There are various ways to make your own pickling weight replacement, small glass dishes work well.) Seal the jar and leave somewhere cool. Your pickled petals will be ready after a few days and will last for a good few years if left unopened.

NOTES

They will start to lose their colour after about a month though. Don't waste the pickling solution after you've eaten the petals, it will make a fantastic salad dressing mixed up with a little oil and seasoning!

Magnolia fritters

These puffy, crispy little magnolia flower fritters are so delicious and just so easy to make! I was completely inspired by the amazing YouTuber Li Ziqi to try battering a magnolia flower and haven't looked back since.

For this recipe we use the whole magnolia flower (without the fluffy leaf sheath) and dip it in tempura batter. It can be slightly tricky to get it to stay flower-shaped so feel free to fritter individual petals if you want an easy life.

MAKES 4

1 egg white
60g (½ cup) plain (all-purpose) flour
80ml (⅓ cup) cold water
Oil, for frying
4 mature magnolia flowers

To serve
Icing (confectioner's) sugar, syrup and shredded magnolia flowers or sweet chilli dip

1. For the batter, beat the egg white until light and frothy, then mix in the flour and enough cold water to make a light, slightly runny batter (you may need a little more or less water).
2. Pour enough oil into a heavy-based pan to come about 5cm (2in) up the sides and place over a medium heat. It's ready when a drop of batter dropped in sizzles and rises to the surface.
3. Take a magnolia flower and release it from its fluffy sheath. It should have a tiny bit of stem left for you to hold on to. (Alternatively, pick off individual petals.)
4. Pop the flower into the batter, giving it a little wiggle to make sure it's completely coated.
5. Use chopsticks to carefully lower the flower into the hot oil. Work with one flower at a time, or a few petals. Be careful not to let the petals stick together, to keep the lovely flower shape – that's why chopsticks are handy.
6. Fry for a few minutes and then flip the flower over and allow to fry for another few minutes on the other side. When the flowers are golden brown and crisp on both sides, they're ready to be served up! Remove from the pan and drain on kitchen towel.
7. Serve them sweet with icing sugar, a little syrup and shredded magnolia flowers, or for a savoury option, plain with a sweet chilli dip.

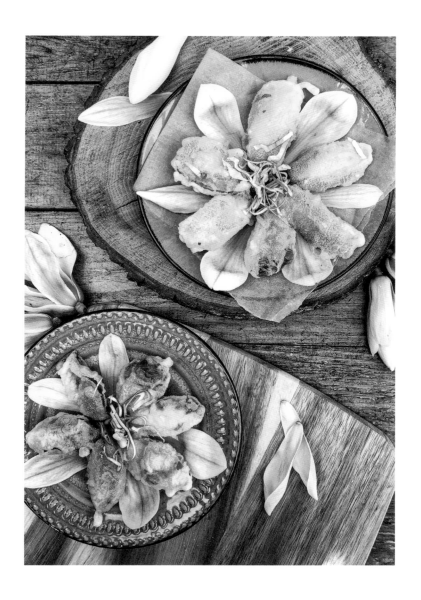

Nettle

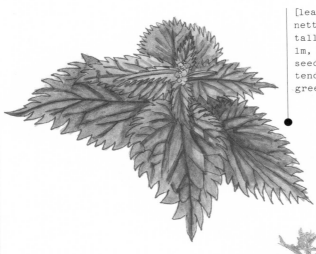

[leaves] Spring nettles are no taller than 1m, have no seeds and have tender, bright green leaves

[leaves] Summer nettles develop tough leaves which we don't cook with, but we can eat the seeds which hang in clusters of green bobbles

[stems] Very tough, green, sometimes with a red or purple tinge. Can grow up to 1.5m (5ft) tall

Foraging notes

The humble nettle is a perfect metaphor for our ever-evolving relationship to plants in the western world. Once relied on as an important source of food, medicine and material, it's now been relegated to the corners of unused fields, forgotten and tarnished. We try to stamp it down, dig it up and throw it aside, unaware of the incredible benefits it can offer us – if we give it a chance!

I'm often asked what my favourite wild ingredient is, and as much as I love gourmet wild mushrooms and ceremonial tree saps, my answer is and always will be nettle. It's an incredible resource and amazingly delicious ingredient that provides all through the year. And the best part is ... it's everywhere and we can all recognise it. It also comes with the promise of a challenge. You probably still have a voice in your head that says, 'don't touch those nettles!' Well, today's the day to take matters into your own (preferably gloved) hands.

The only thing you could get nettle confused with is dead nettle, which has a similar leaf shape but no sting. Thankfully dead nettles are edible too so it's not a problem if you get them mixed up.

To harvest your nettles, wear gloves (washing-up gloves or rubber-dipped gardening gloves are best, as the sting goes through material gloves) and pick only the top 6–8 leaves; these will be the freshest and tastiest. Nettle leaves will get tough and hairy in the summer (see the small illustration on the page opposite) and are best picked in early spring (when they look like the larger illustration on the page opposite). When the seeds appear, the male seeds (the little green bobbles hanging from long strings) can be harvested and used as a superfood sprinkle! They are thought to be a natural stimulant and can give you a little boost of energy when added to food.

Nettle recipes

Nettles need to be cooked (or juiced!) before they're eaten to get rid of those little stinging hairs. When most people try nettles for the first time they boil them for about 10 minutes because they're scared of being stung and then claim with certainty that they've tried nettles and they're gross – no wonder! Try steaming fresh nettle tops for about 4 minutes until they're dark green and wilted and serving with salt and butter and you're sure to be converted to this little green wonder.

Once you've experienced their flavour and feel a little more confident, try nettles in a green soup, a sag aloo, lasagne ... the list goes on! You don't have to stop at savoury recipes either. Try puréeing them down and folding them into cake batter for vibrant green, tasty cakes!

Plant lore, folk medicine & magic

Nettles have been used in so many important ways throughout history, ranging from the practical and mundane to the spiritually significant.

Many cultures, including Europeans and Native Americans, used the fibres from stinging nettle to make sailcloth, sacking, cordage, fishing nets and even clothes. In Denmark, burial shrouds made of nettle fabrics have been discovered that date back to the Bronze Age (3000–2000 BC).

Medicinally they're known to provide relief from arthritis and allergies and in Celtic folklore a large stand of nettles means fairy folk are sure to be living nearby.

Nettle beer

This nettle beer is light, refreshing and perfect on a sunny spring day! It's less like a lager and more like a refreshingly herbal, slightly boozy glass of fizz. Even if brewing isn't something you've done before, this recipe is well worth a go.

MAKES 5 LITRES (8¾ PINTS)

At least 70 nettle tops (the top 6–8 leaves of the stinging nettle)
6 litres (10½ pints) water
500g (1lb 2oz) sugar (any type)
10g (¼oz) brewer's yeast (you can use a beer or wine yeast for this recipe)
Juice of 2 lemons
Thumb-sized piece of fresh ginger, grated (optional)

You will need
1 demijohn or large, sterilised bucket
1 muslin cloth (optional)
Swing top bottles (or use washed large plastic bottles)
Funnel or siphon tube

THE FIRST FERMENT

This is the first ferment. You'll be making your 'wort', which is essentially a tea, plus yeast and sugar. The yeast will eat the sugar, making your nettle beer alcoholic and giving it a beautiful taste.

1. Put the nettle tops into a large pan (you may need to use two) and pour over the water. Bring to the boil, then boil for about 30 minutes until you have a strong nettle tea.
2. Scoop out the cooked nettles and save them for cooking – try making nettle pesto or nettle samosas.
3. Remove the nettle tea from the heat and stir in the sugar until dissolved. Allow your mixture to cool to just above room temperature.
4. Put the brewer's yeast into a small jug and stir up with a little warm water. Pour this into your nettle tea, add the lemon juice and stir. If you want a slightly spicy beer, add the grated ginger to the mix too.
5. Now pour this into your sterilised bucket, or siphon into your demijohn. If you're using a bucket, you'll need to cover it with a muslin cloth.
6. Leave in a warm place for 5–7 days. Keep an eye on the activity. It's ready for bottling when the bubbling has slowed right down.

Recipe continues over the page

THE SECOND FERMENT

This is the second ferment and is all about making your nettle beer fizzy. Now's the time to siphon the beer into your bottles. However, all that fizz means building pressure inside your bottles, which is why plastic bottles are safest. You'll know your brew is fizzy and carbonated by giving the bottle a squeeze (it will be hard) and the sides and bottom of the bottle will bow out. Good-quality swing-top glass bottles are beautiful and the top will pop open if the pressure gets too high. I recommend you don't use glass bottles without a swing top as there is a risk they might explode!

1. Siphon the beer into your bottles. You can try to pour into a funnel but it will be much easier to use a siphon tube, which will only set you back a few pounds.
2. Store your bottles out of the way. If you're using glass, I recommend wrapping them in fabric – just in case!
3. The beer will be ready to drink in around 7 days. Pop open a bottle and taste it; if it's too sweet for you, leave it a few more days. Chill it when it's ready.
4. I like to serve this over ice with lemon slices and mint leaves.
5. Your beer will keep for at least a few months. I've had bottles a year old and they've been delicious.

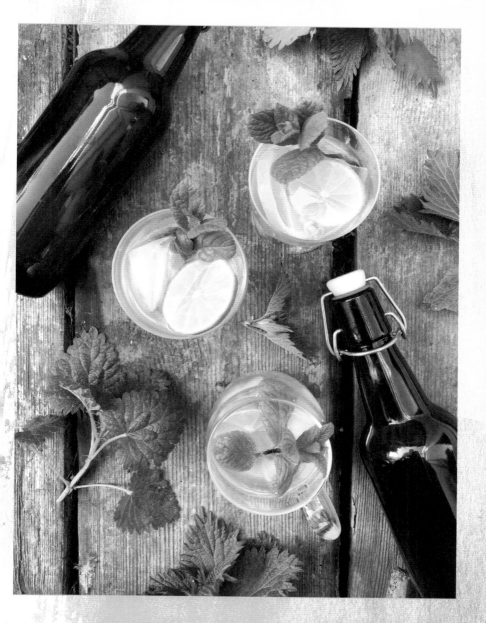

Nettle pakoras

Say hello to little spicy, oh-so-nutritious, crispy pakoras! These are amazing on their own, dipped in chutney or wrapped up in a flatbread with salad.

MAKES ABOUT 8

20 nettle tops
½ white onion, chopped
Thumb-sized piece of fresh ginger, grated
1 tsp ground cumin
1 tsp ground coriander
1 tsp chilli flakes
90g (½ cup) gram (chickpea) flour
2 tbsp rice flour
Oil, for frying

1. Snip the leaves off the nettle tops and steam for 3–4 minutes until dark green and wilted.
2. Add the nettle leaves to a bowl with all the other ingredients (except the oil), then add just enough water to create a really thick batter (I used about 3 tablespoons).
3. Pour a couple of tablespoons of oil into a frying pan and place over a medium heat. Use your hands to mould your pakoras into little flat rounds and shallow-fry in the hot oil for about 3 minutes on each side. Drain on kitchen towel and enjoy immediately.

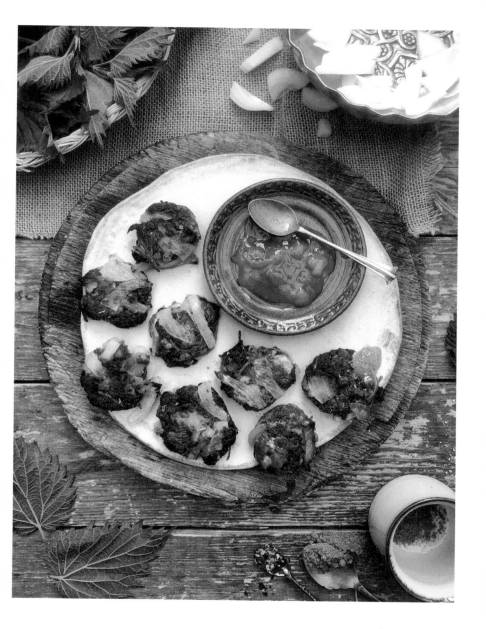

Sticky Weed

[seeds] Small, round, fuzzy green seeds, turning brown with maturity

[flowers] Small flowers with four white petals

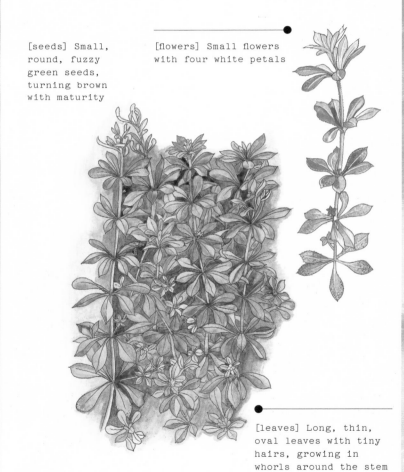

[leaves] Long, thin, oval leaves with tiny hairs, growing in whorls around the stem

Foraging notes

Do you remember walking to school and picking little sticky weeds that were promptly thrown at your friends' school jumpers? Sticky weed is also known as goose grass or cleavers and is not only an excellent game but an incredible edible too!

It's really easy to identify: look for 'whorls' of leaves coming off the stem – 6–7 leaves coming off the stem at the same place, in a star shape – and a very square stem. The closest lookalikes to cleavers are the bedstraw family, which have a similar structure but lack the tiny hook-like hairs on the leaves. This means they won't stick, so your final ID test is to chuck one at the nearest passer-by and make sure it sticks!

Cleavers will grow in huge sticky tangles throughout spring, growing up to 1m (3ft) high. They can be found in hedgerows, alleys, the edges of fields and scrappy corners of gardens. In fact, there's not many places that cleavers don't grow! They'll also make a reappearance in late autumn. Do be careful when you're harvesting cleavers because they stick to other plants as well as jumpers. Pick each stem individually and make sure nothing else is tangled up in them.

Sticky weed recipes

To harvest cleavers, pick the top 7–10cm (2½–4in) and leave any part of the stem that is brown. Cleavers can be used in so many ways. Most simply, you can make a water infusion: just fill up a jar with water, add cleavers and leave in the fridge overnight. In the morning you'll have a lovely detoxifying and tasty infusion. They can also be juiced.

They can be eaten raw but the little hairs make them stick to your throat so to eat them I highly recommend that you always cook them first. I prefer them in recipes where they have been finely shredded or blended.

Plant lore, folk medicine & magic

In Scandinavian folklore the saying goes if you drink an infusion of cleavers for nine weeks, you'll be so beautiful that everyone will fall in love with you! This piece of superstition most likely came from the fact that sticky weed is an amazing spring tonic and detoxifier. If there was ever a superfood, it's this. And our hedgerows are covered in it!

Cleavers are known to aid the lymphatic system, which cleanses the body of toxins. This leads to healthy, glowing skin and gives the immune system a boost too! They're also very high in vitamin C and silica, which is needed for healthy nails, hair and teeth.

Sticky weed and pea soup

This vibrant green soup perfectly encapsulates the freshness of springtime! It's especially good if you can source fresh peas from your local market or garden. The addition of sticky weeds brings a wonderful fresh, almost grassy flavour along with so many health benefits!

SERVES 2

250g (9oz) fresh
   or frozen peas
1 tbsp, plus extra for
   drizzling
Few cubes of butter
1 yellow onion,
   finely chopped
2 celery sticks,
   finely chopped
2 garlic cloves, very
   finely chopped
1 large potato,
   peeled and
   roughly chopped
750ml (3 cups)
   vegetable
   bouillon or broth
2 large bunches of
   cleavers, roughly
   chopped
Juice of ½ lemon
Salt and freshly
   ground black
   pepper

1. If using frozen peas, defrost them by putting in a bowl, pouring over boiling water and letting them sit for 10 minutes before draining.
2. Heat the tablespoon of oil and the butter in a heavy-based pan over a medium-high heat. Add the onion and celery and cook for about 4 minutes, stirring occasionally, until slightly soft and translucent.
3. Add the garlic and cook for another minute, then add the potato and vegetable broth.
4. Cook for about 15 minutes, or until you can push a fork through the potato.
5. Add the cleavers and peas (reserving a few to garnish) and cook for a further minute. Transfer to a blender and blitz until smooth. Taste and add salt, pepper and lemon juice to taste.
6. Serve with a drizzle of olive oil and the reserved peas. This soup is best enjoyed fresh but can also be frozen.

Sticky weed cocktail

This cocktail is perfect for a spring get-together – elegant, light, refreshing and zingy. You'll need a few handfuls worth of cleaver to make the juice for this. If you have a juicer, simply put it through the juicer. If you don't, blend the cleavers in a food processor and then pass through a sieve, pushing down on the plant matter with the back of a spoon to get as much juice as possible. You can experiment with different wild greens too!

SERVES 2

50ml (2fl oz)
  lime juice
70ml (2½fl oz)
  cleaver juice, plus
  a few sprigs to
  garnish
20ml (¾fl oz)
  elderflower
  cordial (see page
  128) or simple
  syrup (optional
  if you prefer a
  sweeter cocktail)
50ml (2fl oz) gin
1 egg white (see
  Note)
Large handful of ice

1. In a cocktail shaker, or a jam jar with a tight-fitting lid if you don't have one, add all of the ingredients apart from the ice.
2. Vigorously shake for around 30 seconds. Your cocktail should look velvety and slightly foamy. Add the ice and continue to shake for another 30 seconds until chilled.
3. Strain the cocktail into two small glasses, garnish with extra sprigs of cleavers or wildflowers and enjoy!

NOTE

If you don't want to use egg white for this recipe, you can use aquafaba, or chickpea water, for the same results.

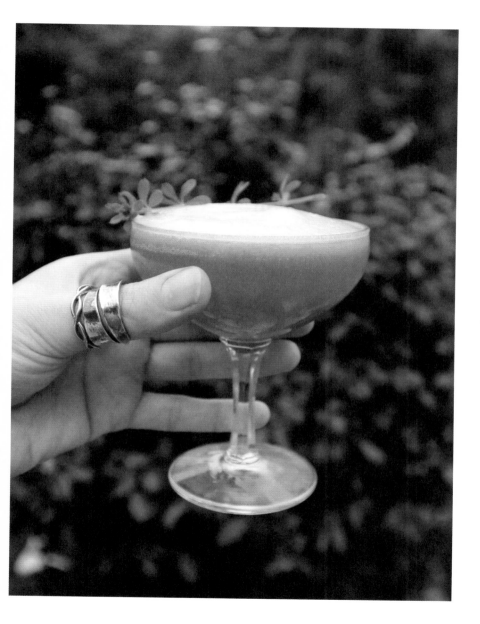

Ground Ivy

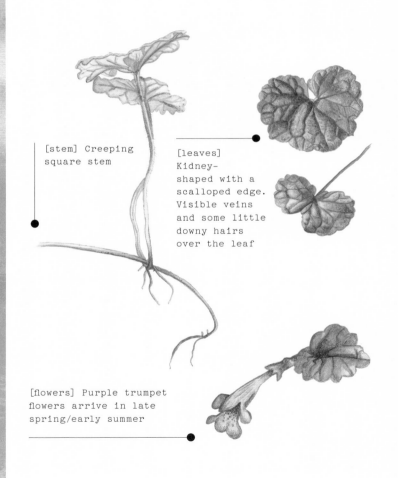

[stem] Creeping
square stem

[leaves]
Kidney-
shaped with a
scalloped edge.
Visible veins
and some little
downy hairs
over the leaf

[flowers] Purple trumpet
flowers arrive in late
spring/early summer

Foraging notes

Ground ivy is a low, creeping plant preferring shady spots, so it can be found lurking at the base of hedgerows and at the edges of fields, and sometimes covering woodland floors. It's a punchy, robust and deeply earthy herb which would have been used in many a medieval kitchen.

It's been used for centuries as a pot herb, a flavouring for ale and as a cure for scurvy. The flavour of ground ivy was well known to our ancestors but has sadly been lost from modern menus. Personally, I think it's time to change that. It's an absolutely delicious ingredient and can be found almost all year round, which makes it a great herb to learn about and use in your wild cooking.

Ground ivy's stems creep along the ground. One leaf should never grow individually from the ground; if you pull it, the whole creeping stem, with lots of other leaves sprouting from it, should come up too. Crush the leaf – does it smell like a mixture of mint and sage? Well, by god, I think you've got it!

NOTE: This plant isn't recommended for anyone who is pregnant or breastfeeding.

Ground ivy recipes

Ground ivy is one of my favourite wild herbs and I use it in the same way as you might use oregano. Chop it down and stir it through salads, make an infused oil, top pizzas and pasta or use to flavour a soup or stew. I mainly use it in savoury dishes, but it can also be used in sweet dishes – why not add a small handful to the dandelion cupcakes, page 84) and cocktails (ground ivy mojito anyone?).

Plant lore, folk medicine & magic

Ground ivy has been used in a myriad of medicinal applications throughout history. Today it is mostly used by medicinal herbalists to treat coughs and congestion and to clear the eyes of infections or styes.

It's also linked with the spring festival of Ostara and was made into a ceremonial wine and incense to please the spring goddesses in pagan times.

Ground ivy and tomato salad

When you pick a few leaves of ground ivy, crush it in your fingers and smell it. You might find it tricky to imagine it in a dish and understand how its flavours might work. But this tomato salad recipe is sure to get you incredibly excited about this little ingredient!

This recipe is best made with organic, heirloom tomatoes bought from the market in a range of colours. You can also add mozzarella and avocado if you like.

SERVES 2

2 large tomatoes
Handful of small
    tomatoes
1 bunch of ground
    ivy leaves
The ends of a stale
    loaf of bread
    (sourdough or
    ciabatta work well)
Good-quality
    olive oil, for
    drizzling
Balsamic vinegar
    (or use elderberry
    and balsamic,
    see page 233), for
    drizzling
Salt and freshly
    ground black
    pepper

1. Roughly chop the large tomatoes, halve the small tomatoes and place in a large salad bowl.
2. Finely chop the ground ivy leaves and add to the bowl, then roughly rip the bread into chunks and add to the bowl too.
3. Drizzle over the olive oil and balsamic vinegar, add a good pinch of salt and pepper and toss to combine.
4. Let your salad sit for at least 15 minutes, ideally somewhere sunny, to allow the juices of the tomatoes to come out and infuse with the ground ivy and soak into the bread.

Ground ivy flatbreads

These soft and fluffy flatbreads are a go-to in my house. They're so quick to make and are great dunked in soup, smothered with toppings like mango chutney and nettle pakoras (see page 64) or as a base for a quick and easy 'pizza' with wild pesto and melted cheese!

MAKES 3 LARGE FLATBREADS

125g (1 cup) self-raising flour, plus extra for dusting
Good pinch of salt
1 tbsp finely chopped ground ivy leaves
200g (⅔ cup) Greek yogurt

1. Add the flour, salt and ground ivy to a large bowl and stir to combine.
2. Add the Greek yogurt and mix until a dough forms.
3. Use your hands to bring the dough together and knead for a moment in the bowl to combine the ingredients. You should have a soft, not sticky dough.
4. Divide the dough into three equal-sized pieces and then roll out on a lightly floured surface until they're roughly 20cm (8in) in diameter.
5. Place a frying pan over a medium heat; when the pan is hot place one of the flatbreads into the pan. Cook for a few minutes on each side, or until the bread has some golden brown spots. Repeat to make the others.
6. Serve hot or cold. These flatbreads are best served fresh and hot but will last for 3 days if wrapped well.

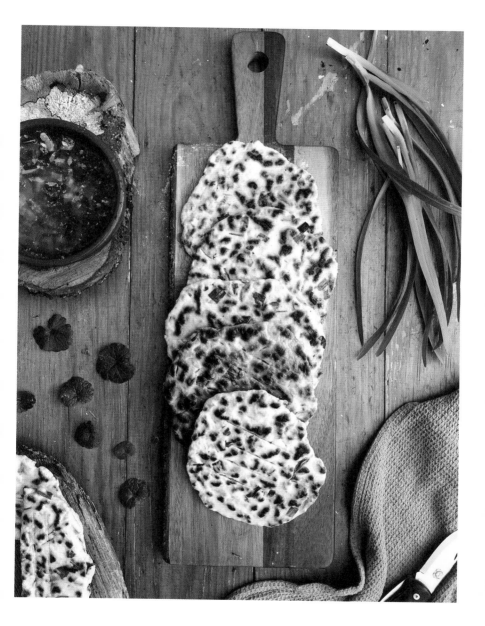

Dandelion

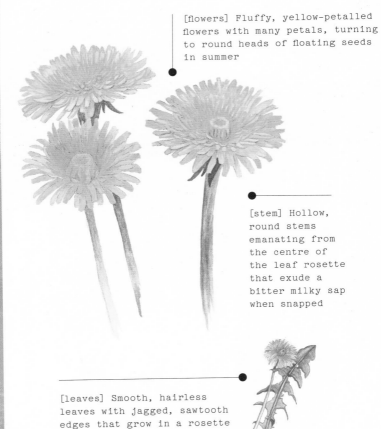

[flowers] Fluffy, yellow-petalled flowers with many petals, turning to round heads of floating seeds in summer

[stem] Hollow, round stems emanating from the centre of the leaf rosette that exude a bitter milky sap when snapped

[leaves] Smooth, hairless leaves with jagged, sawtooth edges that grow in a rosette

Foraging notes

Dandelions are an incredibly underutilised plant. When I see people doing their weeding and throwing handfuls of them on to the compost, I want to give them a dandelion cupcake and a dandelion root latte, so they know what they're missing! They're an incredibly nutritious plant and have been eaten throughout history and across various cultures.

Another great thing about the dandelion is that its closest lookalikes, namely cat's eyes and sow thistles, are also nutritious edibles, so there's no mistaking them for anything that can do you any harm. To make sure you have a true dandelion, look for smooth, hairless leaves and the bitter milky sap that exudes when a leaf or stem is snapped.

Dandelion recipes

Every part of the plant can be eaten: the unopened buds can be pickled like our wild garlic buds (see page 44), the whole flowers can be made into tempura like the magnolia fritters on page 56, and the petals can be used in cakes and pancakes and to make a syrup reminiscent of honey (see page 90, but replace the flowers with dandelion petals). The leaves can be eaten and so can the roots (see page 268).

All parts of the dandelion apart from the petals are very bitter, which is a great sign that you have a powerfully medicinal plant. This may take some getting used to and can be a great advantage in recipes like dandelion root latte (see page 271) but those bitters are well worth getting into your diet! Try some steamed dandelion leaves with butter and salt to start with.

When harvesting dandelion greens, choose the youngest dandelion leaves you can find; they should be light green in colour. If you have some in your garden, pop a flowerpot with a hole in the bottom over the dandelion and return in a few weeks. The dandelion greens will stretch up to reach the light, becoming bigger without becoming any more bitter!

Plant lore, folk medicine & magic

Dandelions feature as a symbol of hope, the coming of summer and the joy of childhood in many folklore tales. They've also been used to take a glimpse into the future throughout our history!

In medieval times a yellow glow on the skin from a dandelion under the chin would be the sign of riches in your future. In the 18th century a dandelion would be held under the chin of a child to predict how sweet and kind they would grow to be.

Dandelions have also long been connected with wishes. When the dandelion petals turn to puffed seeds you can blow on them and they'll turn to fairies, who will fly on the wind and grant you a wish!

Spring greens pie (spanakopita)

This Greek pie is usually made with spinach and feta cheese, but my wild plant-based version uses dandelion greens and tofu. Just as delicious and a perfect springtime treat.

This recipe requires a lot of greens, so feel free to mix in other wild greens or spinach, depending on what's on offer!

MAKES 4 VERY BIG PORTIONS OR 6 SMALLER PORTIONS

1 packet of
  filo pastry (270g)
300g (10oz) fresh
  dandelion greens
2 tbsp olive oil, plus
  extra for greasing
  and brushing
Few cubes of vegan
  butter
1 yellow onion,
  finely chopped
1 leek, finely
  chopped
4 spring onions
  (scallions), finely
  chopped (or
  replace these with
  1 big bunch of
  three-cornered
  leeks)
225g (8oz)
  smoked tofu (or
  use vegan feta)

1. If using frozen filo pastry, take out of the freezer an hour or so before you want to use it.

2. Preheat the oven to 190°C/375°F/gas 5 and place a baking tray in the oven to heat up. Line and grease a deep 20cm (8in) square baking tin.

3. First blanch your dandelion greens; this removes some of the bitterness. Cut any tough bits of stem from the greens (cut up to where the leaf begins to grow) and wash thoroughly. Fill a bowl with iced water. Bring a large saucepan of water to the boil with a good pinch of salt. When boiling, add the dandelion greens and cook for 3 minutes. Transfer the greens straight into the bowl of iced water. Drain thoroughly, squeezing out the excess water, then place on kitchen towel to air dry.

4. Heat the oil in a large saucepan with the butter. When hot, add the onions and leek and sauté, stirring regularly for about 10 minutes over a medium-high heat until slightly caramelised and golden brown.

5. Add the spring onions, crumble in the smoked tofu and cook for another 4 minutes. Add the herbs and spinach, vegetable stock paste and salt and pepper to taste. Cook for another 2 minutes, or until all the spinach has wilted down. Add the blanched dandelion leaves and cook for a further minute until there is no moisture in the bottom of the pan.

Recipe continues over the page

Small bunch of fresh
    dill (or use yarrow,
    see page 152)
Small bunch of
    fresh parsley
Leaves from
    a few sprigs of
    fresh mint
300g (10oz) spinach
1 tbsp vegetable
    stock paste
Salt and freshly
    ground black
    pepper
Sesame seeds,
    for sprinkling

6. To keep your pastry moist, unroll it and cover it with
    a damp cloth. Place one sheet of filo on to the baking
    tin and oil it. Repeat for the next five layers of filo,
    turning the tin 90 degrees between each layer so
    you cover all four sides of the tin. Don't worry if it
    overhangs the edges.

7. Pour your filling into the baking tin and flatten with
    a spoon. Now begin to fold the overhanging pastry over
    to form a lid, brushing each layer with oil as you fold it
    down. You shouldn't be able to see the filling. If you have
    folded all the pastry in and you still can, add more layers
    of pastry, oiling as you go and folding each layer in on
    itself. Score the pastry where you will cut it into squares,
    then sprinkle with sesame seeds.

8. Place the baking tin on the preheated baking tray and
    bake for 25–30 minutes, or until the top is golden brown.

9. You can serve your spring greens pie hot or cold. It's
    delicious with a herby yogurt dip!

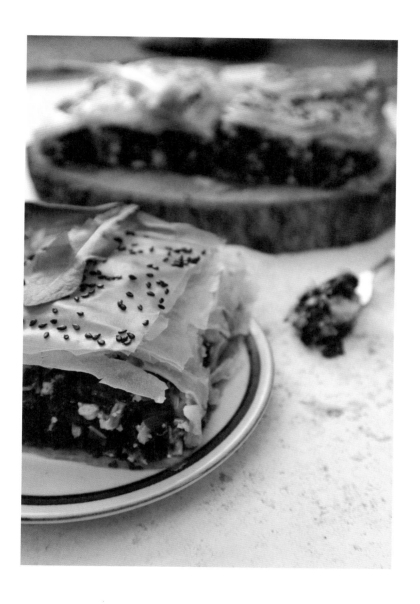

Dandelion cupcakes

These soft, fluffy, herbal little cakes of sunshine and joy are one of my favourite ways to use dandelion petals – they were such a winner in my house during lockdown!

MAKES 6 CUPCAKES

Approx. 30–40 dandelion heads
75g (3oz) butter, softened
75g (3oz) caster (superfine) sugar
1 egg
1 tsp vanilla extract
75g (scant ½ cup) self-raising flour
4 tbsp milk
1 tbsp chopped fresh herbs, such as ground ivy or thyme

To decorate
1 tbsp marmalade
1 tbsp icing (confectioner's) sugar
Few dandelion petals and ground ivy flowers

1. First process your dandelion heads by picking off the petals and discarding any green part of the flower, which will be very bitter. You will need enough to fill ¼ cup.
2. Preheat the oven to 180°C/350°F/gas 4 and line a cupcake tin with six paper cases.
3. Cream together the butter and sugar until pale and creamy.
4. Add the egg, vanilla, flour and milk and mix until you have a smooth batter. Fold in the dandelion petals and chopped herbs.
5. Spoon the mixture into the paper cases, then bake in the oven for 20 minutes, or until the tops are golden and springy to the touch. Allow to cool on a wire rack.
6. While the cakes are in the oven, make the icing by mixing the marmalade and icing sugar together until smooth.
7. Spread the icing over the cooled cupcakes, then decorate with extra dandelion petals and ground ivy flowers.

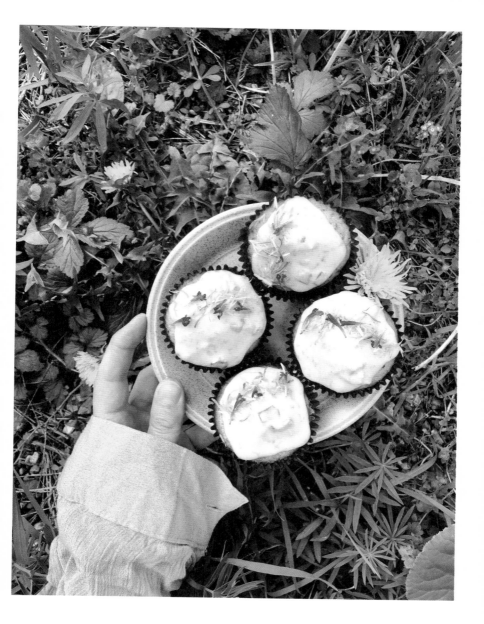

Lilac

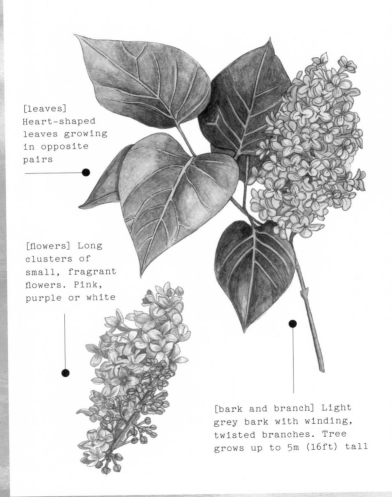

[leaves]
Heart-shaped
leaves growing
in opposite
pairs

[flowers] Long
clusters of
small, fragrant
flowers. Pink,
purple or white

[bark and branch] Light
grey bark with winding,
twisted branches. Tree
grows up to 5m (16ft) tall

Foraging notes

When spring is reaching a glittering crescendo, and long sunny days have begun to bless us, pretty plumes of delicate little lilac flowers bloom in long clusters, looking like masses of elegant, floral-scented party poppers, released from a bushel of heart-shaped leaves.

Just a few of these clusters can bring a huge dose of joy to so many sweet treats and I often wonder why lilac water isn't as popular as rose water. As with all of our fragrant, sweet wildflowers, lilacs make amazing jam, syrup, icing and tea, as well as being a beautiful garnish for desserts and cakes.

You may notice that other garden flowers, such as buddleia, have a similar structure, with pink or purple long clusters of flowers. These lookalikes all have long, thin leaves, rather than heart-shaped leaves. You can also tell lilac with a close inspection of the flowers, which are long and tubular with four petals.

Lilac recipes

The only part of the lilac that is edible is the flower. Before making any of these recipes, you should pick off the individual flowers before transforming them into delicious works of edible art!

Plant lore, folk medicine & magic

Lilacs have inspired people with their beauty and allure throughout history. In Greek mythology lilacs came into being when a forest nymph called Syringa ran through the woods to avoid the keen advances of a suitor. He chased her through the woods, so, with nowhere to hide, she turned herself into a lilac bush.

Lilac is thought to have calming and soothing qualities so works in a similar way to rose water for skincare. As an astringent it helps to draw out impurities and calm redness. You might also find herbalists using an infusion of lilac to help soothe burns and itching.

'Lilac is though to have calming and soothing qualities.'

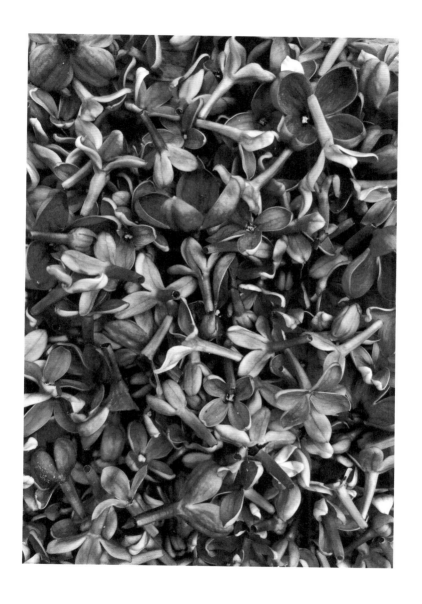

Lilac honey

You can use this honey to stir into herbal teas, bringing a beautiful floral touch, to make honey cakes, baklava or – my favourite way to use it – to drizzle generously on buttered crumpets! Don't forget to try it with savoury dishes too. It's particularly good on a goat's cheese and walnut salad.

I really urge you to go and buy some local honey for this recipe; local beekeepers do such important work for the environment and they deserve our support.

MAKES 1 JAR

50g (2oz) fresh
   lilac flowers
1 jar of local honey

1. Take your fresh lilac flowers and pick them off the stem, ensuring you have only the colourful flower.
2. Take a sterilised jam jar, the same size or slightly bigger than your jar of honey, and sprinkle around a quarter of the flowers into the jar. Top up a quarter of the way with honey (give it a stir if you see air bubbles at this stage) and repeat the process until the jar is full.
3. Leave the jar in a cool dark place for 1 week, stirring every few days, or until your honey tastes fragrant.
4. Over time, your flowers with float to the top which is fine – they are still infusing!
5. Your lilac honey is now ready to enjoy. I personally leave the flowers in and enjoy them along with the honey, but you can scoop them out of the jar if you don't want the floral taste to get any stronger.
6. Your lilac honey will last for 3 months in a cool, dark place. If you'd like to make a lilac honey that will last all year, dry your lilac flowers before making this recipe.

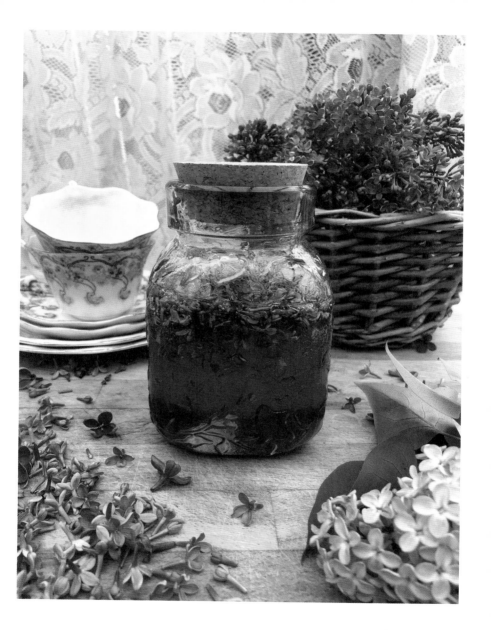

Lilac, lemon and rhubarb jars

These little pudding jars are a glorious jumble of all things springtime! Fresh, vibrant rhubarb, tangy lemon and sweet and perfumed lilac come together beautifully here.

SERVES 4

For the lemon yogurt
400g (14oz) tub of plain oat or almond yogurt
Flowers from 2 sprigs of lilac (approx. 50g/2oz)
150g (5oz) lemon curd

For the crumb
1½ tbsp coconut oil
100g (3½oz) oats
50g (2oz) blanched almonds, roughly chopped
½ tsp ground cinnamon
2 tbsp maple syrup

For the rhubarb compote
4 sticks of forced rhubarb (approx. 300g/10oz)
2 tbsp caster (superfine) sugar

Crystallised lilac flowers (see page 97), to decorate

1. The night before, put the lilac flowers into the yogurt and stir to infuse overnight.
2. In the morning, make the crumb. Preheat the oven to 160°C/325°F/gas 3 and line a baking tray with baking parchment. Melt the coconut oil in a saucepan, then remove from heat and add the remaining ingredients. Stir until the oats are coated. Pour into the lined tray and bake for 15–20 minutes, or until golden brown around the edges. Remove from the oven, press down with the back of a spatula and leave in the tray until completely cooled.
3. Increase the oven temperature to 180°C/350°F/gas 4.
4. Cut the rhubarb into 5cm (2in) long pieces. Cut any thick pieces you have in half lengthways so they're all similar size. Place in a deep baking tray with 100ml (3½fl oz) water and sprinkle with the caster sugar. Cover with foil and bake for 10–15 minutes, or until the rhubarb is tender. Once cooked, set aside until cooled.
5. Remove the yogurt from the fridge and swirl through the lemon curd for a rippled effect.
6. To assemble, take four small jars or glasses and break some crumb to sit at the bottom. Next add some rhubarb and then top with yogurt. Add more rhubarb, a drizzle of rhubarb juice and top with crystallised lilac flowers (see the method for crystallised violets on page 97).

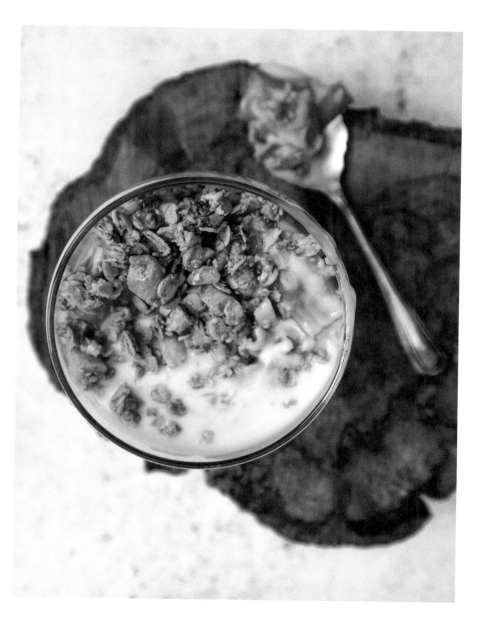

Wild Violet

[flowers] Blue, purple
or white with two
broad upward-facing
petals and three
thinner downward-
facing petals

[stem] Swan-
like neck,
which droops
down before
it displays a
flower

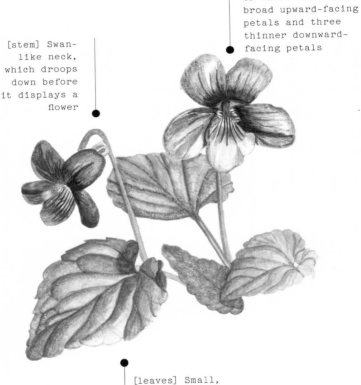

[leaves] Small,
hairless, heart-shaped
leaves

Foraging notes

Wild violets can often be found in abundance as a lawn weed, or completely covering areas of woodland floor. They like shady spaces and can be hard to spot, as the flowers face downwards. Look for a little glint of purple among heart-shaped leaves.

In this book I'm offering a few recipes which will make the most of just a few wild violets, but if you come across an abundance of them, you'll be able to make colour-changing potions, cocktails and cordials. If you make a violet flower syrup it will be purple, but pour in a little lemon juice ... and it will turn pink! If you really want to try making one of these colour-changing potions but can't find enough wild violets, you can also try it with blue butterfly pea flowers, which you can buy online.

Wild violet recipes

Both the leaves and flowers of the wild violet are edible. Pick the young leaves to add to a wild salad or pick a very small amount of wild violets to use in very special recipes. Or you can just enjoy them, and listen to stories about them.

Plant lore, folk medicine & magic

Greek legend told of a nymph named Io, who was beloved by Zeus. To hide her from Hera, his wife, Zeus changed Io into a white cow. When Io wept over the taste and texture of the coarse grass, Zeus created dainty, sweet-smelling violets for her to eat.

In Christianity, the violet symbolises modesty and humility, as the flower hides its beauty under its downward-facing petals, which is why it became the flower of the Virgin Mary. One ancient tale tells us that all violets were once white, until Mary watched her son die on the cross. As she was overcome with anguish, all the violets in the world turned purple to echo her mourning. Maybe that's why purple is still associated with mourning!

Crystallised wild violets

These crystallised violets are super-simple to make. Pick your wild violets, paint with egg white (for a vegan alternative you could use aquafaba, or the liquid from a tin of chickpeas) and dust with caster sugar – coconut sugar makes a nice alternative for a healthier sweet. Leave them on a flat surface to dry for about an hour. They will be delicate and crisp and taste like the most delicious Parma Violet you've ever had. Enjoy them as they are or use them to decorate pretty iced cupcakes. They'll last in an airtight container lined with kitchen towel for up to 2 months.

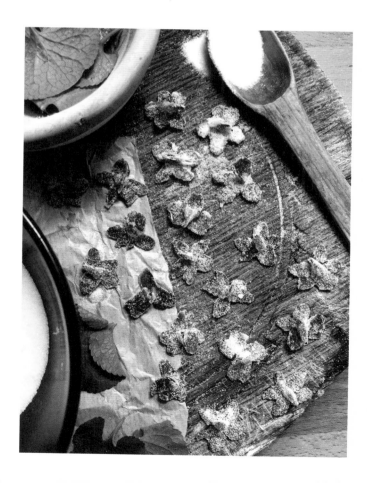

Wildflower biscuits

These rolled biscuits are a fantastic way to showcase the beauty and delicacy of the wildflowers on offer in spring. Choose wildflowers in a range of different sizes, shapes and colours for some truly charming biscuits.

MAKES 15 BISCUITS

100g (3½oz) unsalted butter, at room temperature
100g (½ cup) caster (superfine) sugar
½ tsp vanilla extract
1 medium egg
200g (generous 1½ cups) plain (all-purpose) flour, plus a little extra for dusting
Selection of edible wildflowers, e.g. wild violets, lilac flowers, ground ivy flowers, dandelion petals
Sprinkle of granulated sugar, to decorate

1. Preheat the oven to 200°C/400°F/gas 6 and line a baking tray with baking parchment.

2. Cream the butter and sugar together until pale, light and fluffy – you can do this in a bowl with a wooden spoon or use an electric mixer, if you have one.

3. In a separate bowl or cup, stir the vanilla extract into the egg with a fork. Pour about three-quarters of this mixture into your butter and sugar mixture (keep the remainder to glaze the biscuits before they go in the oven), then add the flour. Use a wooden spoon to mix together until a dough forms.

4. Lightly dust your work surface with flour and roll out your dough – you want it to be the thickness of two pound coins.

5. Use a biscuit cutter to mark out biscuit shapes in the dough, but don't push them into the dough just yet. Lay the wild flowers over the biscuits; when they're all in position, roll again, very lightly, to press them in slightly.

6. To fix your flowers and ensure they don't burn, use your leftover egg mixture to brush over all the flowers and tops of the biscuits, then cut out the biscuits and transfer to your baking sheet.

7. Bake the biscuits for 8–10 minutes until lightly golden – keep an eye on them, to make sure the edges don't brown. Transfer to a wire rack to cool and sprinkle with a little granulated sugar while they are still warm.

8. These will keep for about 4 days in an airtight container.

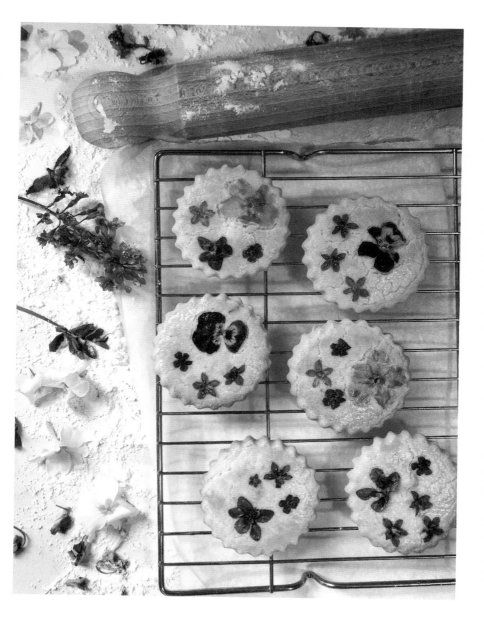

Spring Self-care

With an abundance of wild greens, flowers and sunny days on offer, sometimes a walk in nature is all the self-care we need in at this time of year. Drinking in the sounds of the birds, feeling the sun's warmth on our faces and allowing the colours and light to wash over us feels like bliss after the long, cold winter and is, of course, truly nourishing for the awakening soul.

Entering spring can often feel like awakening from hibernation. The change in pace can at times be overwhelming so remember to echo nature: wake up slowly and allow yourself to adjust to the changing seasons with kindness and patience. Fill your body with nourishing foods and welcome a new phase of the year without judgement or expectation.

Spring is a time to realise new intentions and to start new chapters. Take time to consider what new energies and activities you might like to welcome into your life.

'Echo nature: wake up slowly and allow yourself to adjust to the changing seasons.'

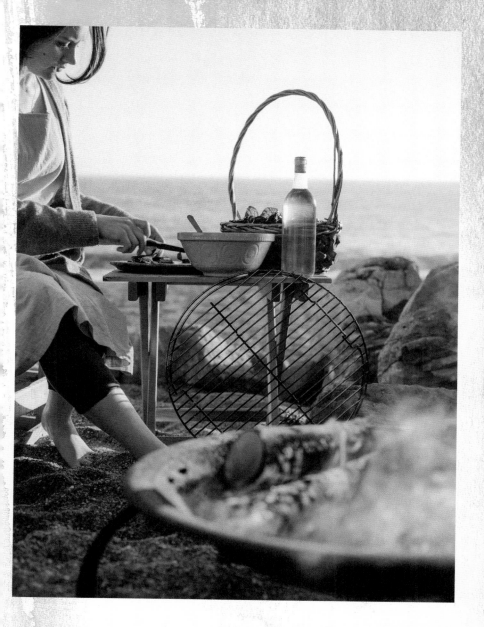

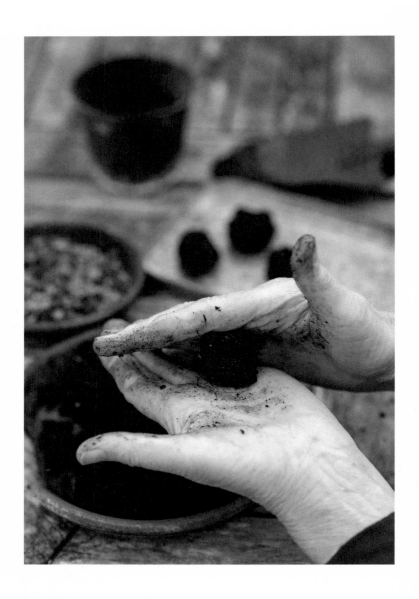

Spring Rituals

Make wild seed bombs

These wild seed bombs are an absolute pleasure to make and have their roots in rebellious acts of guerrilla gardening. They originated in Japan where they were known as 'Earth Dumplings', eventually making their way to the US, where they were thrown onto abandoned plots of land and bare, unloved roadsides by those wanting to help biodiversity and were tired of waiting for the government to do it.

Scattering them in your garden, local meadows, hedgerows and empty urban areas will bring a little extra life and diversity to the land and – even better – attract pollinators. Make sure never to introduce anything other than native wildflowers, and don't seed bomb agricultural land or conservation sites, as it may go against existing conservation plans.

Remember that you can collect your own wild seeds in autumn to make these wild seed bombs (see page 236). You can also buy native wild seed online or you can attend a 'seed swapping event'. These usually take place in February and are a great opportunity to meet other plant lovers.

In a bowl, mix 1 cup of plain (all-purpose) flour and 3 cups of seed compost together until combined. Add ¼ cup of native wildflower seed and gently fold through the mixture. Begin adding water while gently combining with your hands. Add just enough water so that the mixture begins forming clumps – you don't want it too wet. Mix well and start rolling roughly golf ball-sized balls.

Leave the balls out for 24 hours to dry, then go out to spread your seed bombs in empty spaces. The best time to do this is just before it's forecast to rain! If you have a particular area in mind, it's a good idea to get an idea of what seed will work well there.

For sunny spaces try chamomile, buttercup, poppies, bird's foot trefoil, marigold, cornflower, hollyhock, common spotted orchid, wild thyme, red clover. For shady woodland areas try foxgloves, honesty, sweet woodruff, betony, selfheal.

Celebrate Ostara

In the northern hemisphere, the spring equinox takes place every year on either 20 or 21 March. It's the day that both night and day are equal in length, meaning that we are in perfect balance. It's the turning point which will take us into the brighter half of the year and so, naturally, is a time to celebrate!

Spring equinox is also known as Ostara, who was celebrated by pagans as the goddess of dawn and fertility. Ostara was also known as Eostre, which eventually became Easter.

By looking back to Ostara, and celebrating spring equinox in a more traditional way than the modern habit of giving chocolate eggs, we embrace what's important: our gratitude and connection to the turning of the wheel, the change of the seasons and living in harmony with nature.

Now is a wonderful time to enjoy spring feasts made from sustainably foraged ingredients. Decorate your home with bright colours and give thanks to nature by planting plenty of seeds to help as much new life as possible bloom. Remember that plenty of insects and animals will be on the hunt for sustenance at this time too, and will be bringing new life of their own into the world. Do what you can to help them enjoy the bounty of nature – leave out birdseed, watch out for nests when you are foraging and leave piles of twigs and woodland debris undisturbed.

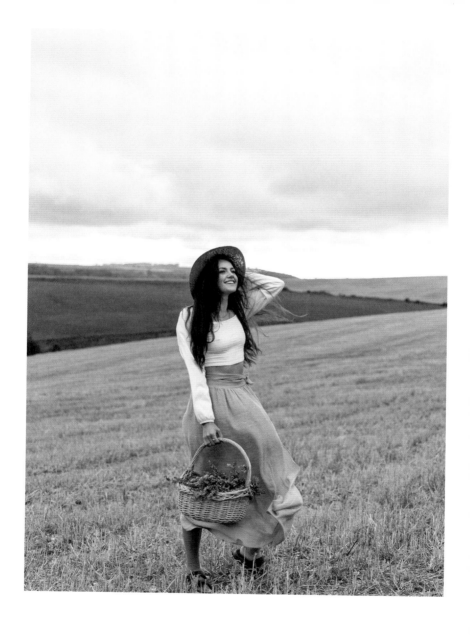

Summer

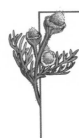

Summer is, and has always been, a time for festivities, celebrations and joy. As the wheel of the year turns, the days get longer and the sun warms the air, stirring up an unexplainable shared excitement. We echo nature, even if we do so unconsciously; the flowers bloom, and so do we!

The grass grows tall and colour fills in the gaps between once bare branches. Wild roses crawl over the hedgerows and decorate the thorny heights of the blackthorn as if someone's sprinkled them with pink confetti. Honeysuckle bursts open triumphantly, singing of sweet nectar and inviting busily pollinating bees from their hives.

The meadows now seem full to bursting, the tall grass dances with wildflowers and builds itself into a kingdom for insects. As you carefully step through, you're greeted by the chirping, buzzing and whirring of life beneath your feet. Butterflies flutter upwards and skip from blade to blade and little grasshoppers leap to the side.

Even our urban areas flourish with floral blooms and seem to have invited nature to stay for a while. Huge bushels of lavender proudly stand tall and lean over stone walls of neighbours' gardens, inviting you to rub your fingers over their purple buds and delight in their sweet and nurturing smell. Bright, sunshine-yellow nasturtium flowers begin blooming and awaken the taste buds with their peppery flavours.

Summer is a time to invite the lightness, beauty and joy so easily observed in our wild spaces into your body and into your home.

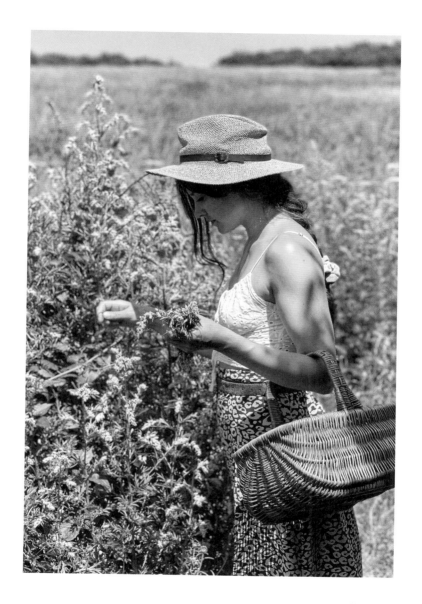

Foraging in Summer

There is an incredible range of goodies to be foraged for in summer. In June the meadows and parks begin to offer up spectacularly fragranced wildflowers and herbs. July brings huge blooms of elderflowers, perfect for champagnes and cordials. By the time August rolls around the hedgerows will already be bursting with ripe fruits like blackberries and elderberries and my kitchen transforms into a jam-making factory. (And that's without even touching on nature's coastal offerings and selection of summer mushrooms!)

Medicinal herbs

Many of our wonderfully mild spring greens become very powerful and bitter in summer, but that doesn't mean we can't make use of them any more.

Some greens, like cleavers and wild garlic, might disappear completely but others will stick around and develop their flavours. Greens like yarrow and mugwort, which were very mild in spring and could be added to salad bowls without a second thought, are now astringent and strong in flavour. We can still use them, however; firstly we can use them as a herb for flavouring, rather than as the main green element in our dishes and salads, and secondly they are now considered potent medicinal herbs.

Medicinal herbs are always close by, if we know where to look. As foragers, we're consuming ancient medicines all the time, whether knowingly or not.

I've seen plenty of people look at me sceptically when I start talking about using wild herbs as medicines but I think it's enough to remind them that very many of the pharmaceutical

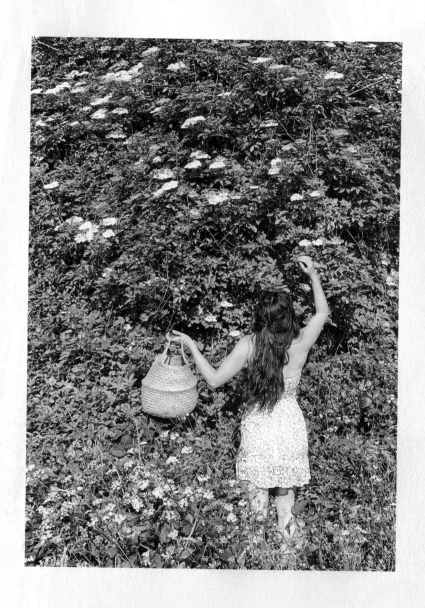

drugs on sale today are derived from plants (see page 15). This is more astounding still when you consider only a tiny fraction of all plants have ever been scientifically tested for medicinal uses. The funding simply isn't there.

Those same sceptics might say, 'scientific testing is the only way to really know if a medicine works'. But our medicinal plants have been tested, time and time again. Native people, whose medicinal knowledge is passed down, would have only used the medicines which worked. Generation after generation have tested our plant medicines.

Wild herbs can be used externally – by infusing with oil and making into balms and lotions for an array of skincare issues – or taken internally, simply by adding a handful to your salad or by making an infusion or a tincture.

Remember that wild herbs are powerful medicines. This does mean that if you're pregnant, or taking medication, you should do your research before consuming wild herbs.

Although we don't have the space in this book to discuss medicinal herbs at length, here are just a few of the medicinal uses for the herbs in this chapter:

YARROW (used externally)
wound staunching, antimicrobial, antibacterial
YARROW (used internally)
menstruation (to correct both heavy, painful and late periods), reducing fever
MUGWORT (used externally)
muscle relaxing, insect repellent

MUGWORT (used internally) lucid dreaming, aids the liver, aids digestion, calms the nervous system
PLANTAIN (used externally)
relief for stings and insect bites, cleaning wounds
PLANTAIN (used internally)
relieves coughs and sore throats, hay fever and allergies

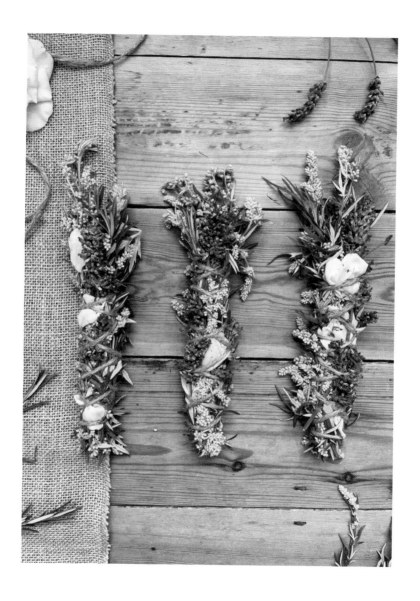

Fruits

Many wild fruits ripen in the autumn, but late summer is a brilliant time for damsons, elderberries, rowan berries, bilberries and wild strawberries in particular. Dog walks become a little slower as we stop to munch blackberries along the hedgerows and many a sunny day is spent in the cool woodland, picking bilberries with purple-stained fingers.

Fruits have, of course, been eaten throughout history, whether fresh, dried or made into wine. Archaeologists even found evidence of cranberry wine in a container made of birch bark in a Bronze Age grave in Denmark.

Foraging for fruits has some excellent benefits over shop-bought. Firstly, the fruits we buy at the supermarket are very often genetically modified varieties, created to be as big and shiny and visually appealing as possible. However, with all that attention given to their looks, they end up lacking a lot of substance. Not only are they considerably less flavourful than their wild counterparts, but also lacking in nutritional density. Secondly, you can pick your fruits at precisely the right time. Supermarket fruits are usually picked too early, so they never ripen naturally and are often sprayed with pesticides or fungicides. While foraging, you can locate your fruit tree and keep visiting it until those fruits are perfectly soft!

There's also a lot of mysticism, symbolism and folklore in the world of fruits! For example, according to Celtic and Manx folklore, the first blackberries of the season should be left for the fairy folk. Failing to do so will result in the rest of the berries you pick being full of grubs!

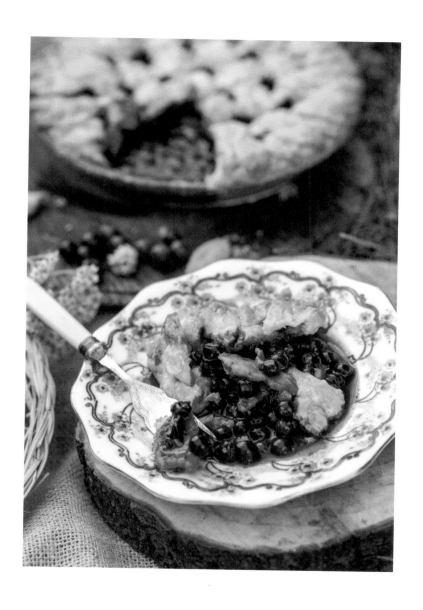

Rose

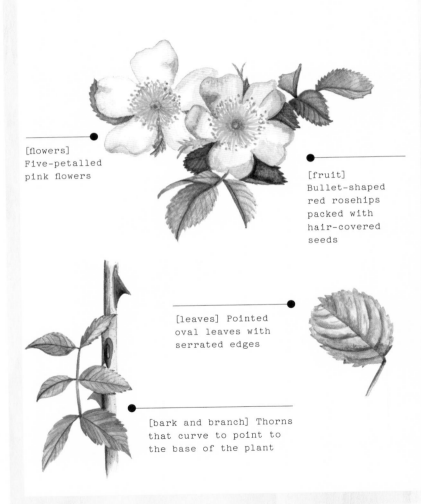

[flowers]
Five-petalled
pink flowers

[fruit]
Bullet-shaped
red rosehips
packed with
hair-covered
seeds

[leaves] Pointed
oval leaves with
serrated edges

[bark and branch] Thorns
that curve to point to
the base of the plant

Foraging notes

There's nothing like the heady smell of roses floating on a summer breeze. It carries with it an unrivalled air of romanticism and a depth of meaning that doesn't have to be recognised to be influential. The scent of rose brings elegance to anything it touches.

Although we are of course focusing on wild magic in this book, I would really recommend harvesting unsprayed garden roses when you want to use them for their petals. This is because wild roses only have five petals, whereas garden roses have many more, so collecting these means we'll end up leaving a lot more for the pollinators.

When picking rose petals, remember that pollinators use the colourful petals to find their way to the stamen, which holds the pollen. By leaving at least one petal on the flower, the pollinators will still be able to find their way to the sweet stuff!

To capture the essence of the rose in summer you can either use your petals to make a jam or syrup, or you can make rose water. This can be done in so many ways, from following the steps in my rose water recipe (see page 120), to simply adding rose petals to a jar of water and leaving it on a sunny windowsill, in the same way so many of us did as children when 'making perfume'. Once you have your rose water, you can use it in all manner of ways!

Later in the year, the rose will produce its berries, or 'hips' (see page 262). These little red berries are bursting with vitamin C and are amazing for making jams and syrups.

Rose recipes

As with all wildflowers, there are many ways to introduce rose to your dishes. A sprinkle of rose petals makes for a wonderful garnish and, crystalised, they make beautiful wild sweets. But when I'm working with rose, I usually make rosewater.

Rose water has been around for thousands of years and is thought to originate from what is now Iran. It has a surprising number of health benefits, including anti-inflammatory properties, which may help to soothe irritated skin and symptoms of eczema and reduce redness. Recent studies have even suggested it could help to reduce depression and anxiety.

You can use it in self-care recipes: as a cooling and soothing facial toner, as a herbal pillow spritz or as a natural air freshener. It's also great in recipes such as cakes and biscuits, in rice dishes, any dish with honey and pistachios, or in iced tea or cocktails!

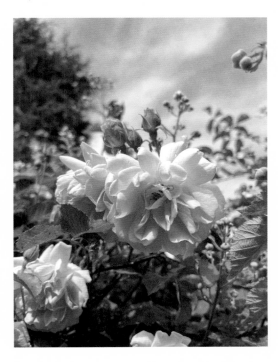

Plant lore, folk medicine & magic

In England, France and other European cultures, it is seen as bad luck and an omen of ill-fate if a petal falls from the rose while you're cutting it or gifting it to someone. It's thought that sleeping with a rosehip under your pillow will protect from bad dreams.

In Greek mythology, the rose is strongly associated with Aphrodite, the goddess of love. It's said that when she came into being, she rose from the froth of the sea. When the sea foam fell to the earth, white roses grew. Later in her life she would fall deeply in love with a mortal named Adonis, and when he was fatally wounded by a wild boar, she ran to him. On her journey, she pricked her foot on a thorn and stained a white rose red with her blood. This was the first red rose to ever be seen on earth. These ancient stories echo the modern symbolism of the white rose for innocence and the red rose for passionate love.

Rose water

Your rose water will be the base of many recipes to come so you want the scent to be just right! You can get a good idea of what the rose water will smell like by smelling the roses that you plan to use before picking them. Red and pink roses usually have a strong and traditional rose fragrance, but you could also try white and yellow roses for more of a unique fragrance, with citrussy, vanilla undertones.

MAKES APPROX. 200ML (GENEROUS ¾ CUP)

Petals from
4–5 blooms of (unsprayed) fragrant garden roses, or from around 40 dog roses
Approx. 500ml (2 cups) water
1 tray of ice cubes

1. Put the petals into a saucepan, then place a medium-sized bowl, such as a cereal bowl, in the centre of the pan, so that it is sitting nestled among the rose petals. Make sure there is a gap of at least a few centimetres around the edge of the bowl.
2. Now carefully pour the water on top of the rose petals (don't get any in the bowl in the centre).
3. Place the pan over a high heat and bring the water to the boil. As soon as you can see small bubbles in the water, reduce the heat to a simmer.
4. Put a lid on the saucepan, but upside down, then fill the concave saucepan lid with ice cubes. As the water boils in the pan the steam will rise, hit the cold lid, run down to the centre of the lid and drip into the bowl. As and when the ice melts during the process, top it up with fresh ice. Keep going until you have almost no water left in the pan (keep an eye on it as you don't want the saucepan to boil dry) and the bowl is full of rose water!
5. Allow the whole thing to cool (don't try to lift the hot bowl out – you'll probably lose your rose water). Pour the rose water into a sterilised spray bottle or glass jar and keep in the fridge for up to 2 months.

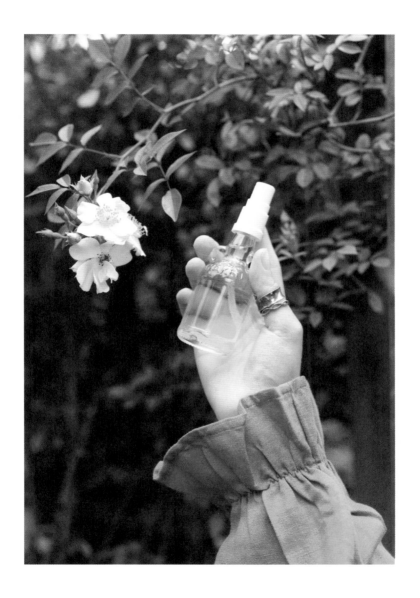

Rose and chocolate ice lolly

These ice lollies are astoundingly good and perfectly refreshing on a hot summer day. They were inspired by the lovely Leanne at Wild Food Stories who wanted to make her son's favourite ice lollies (can you guess which brand?) from wild ingredients!

My take on these lollies is made with a creamy elderflower cordial and a raspberry purée flavoured with rose water. The ends are dipped in dark chocolate and rolled in a mixture of dried rose petals, dried chamomile flowers and candied rosehips, although you could top yours with anything you like – how about dried nuts, coconut flakes or fresh flower petals?

MAKES 4 ICE LOLLIES

50g elderflower cordial (see page 128)
150ml milk (I use oat milk)
4 edible flowers (I used oxeye daisies but you could use elderflowers or rose petals)
200g fresh or frozen raspberries
1-2 tbsp rose water
100g good-quality dark chocolate
100g mixed chosen toppings (dried or fresh edible flower petals, chopped dried nuts, fruit or coconut flakes)

1. Make up a batch of elderflower cordial but using plant milk instead of water; you want the ratio of cordial to plant milk to be the same as you'd make for a glass of elderflower cordial.
2. Pour into ice-lolly moulds so that the moulds are about two-thirds full, then pop it in the freezer.
3. After a few hours, push some edible flowers or rose petals into the moulds, so that half of them are submerged in the icy liquid. Return to the freezer for at least 6 hours.
4. Whizz up your raspberries in a blender until you have a purée, then stir in the rose water to taste. Fill up the top third of each ice-lolly mould, pressing the flowers or petals against the sides of the mould so that they show through when frozen. Return to the freezer for a further 6 hours until fully frozen.
5. Melt the dark chocolate, either in a heatproof bowl in the microwave or using a bain marie. Remove the lollies from the moulds and dip the top third of each lolly into the chocolate.
6. Put your chosen toppings on to a plate and dip the chocolate-coated lollies in them. Return to the freezer to allow the chocolate to set.

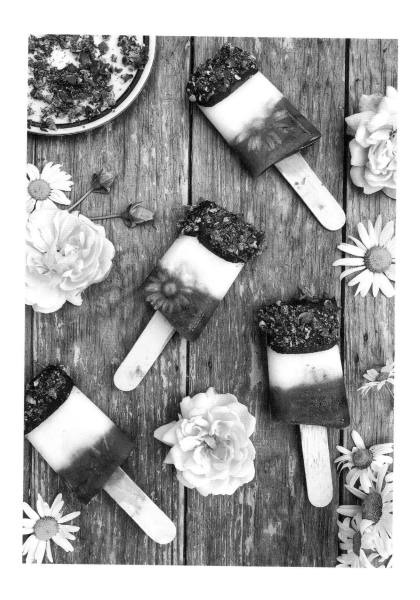

Elderflower

[flowers] Flat, white sprays of
flowers are all the same size and
have obvious yellow stamens

[fruit]
See page 228

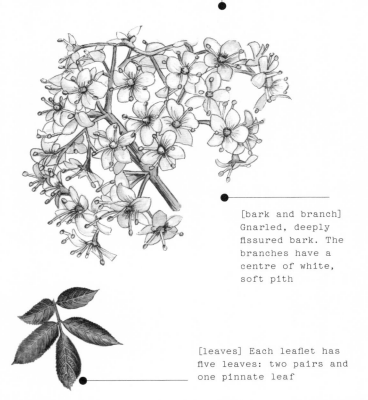

[bark and branch]
Gnarled, deeply
fissured bark. The
branches have a
centre of white,
soft pith

[leaves] Each leaflet has
five leaves: two pairs and
one pinnate leaf

Foraging notes

If you see me in the fields on a summer day, giddily picking white blooms of flowers from gnarled trees, with a yellow pollen-tipped nose and a giddy look upon my face, it's elderflower season.

The elderflower portrays summer perfectly, with its sweet and alluring scent, its lacy blooms which are best picked on a still and sunny day and the array of wonderful celebration dishes that can be made from them, from Turkish delight, pavlovas, biscuits, curds, cakes and crème brûlées to cordials and cocktails. All wonderful, and most as simple as adding some freshly made elderflower cordial to your favourite recipe!

The elder is said to be a tree that gives us what we need, when we need it and has been used as a healing plant dating back as far as 400 BC, when Hippocrates, the 'Father of Medicine', called the elder tree his 'medicine chest'. Tea made with the flowers has traditionally been used as a brilliant summer time remedy for hay fever sufferers, while the berries that come along a little later in the year are an immunity-boosting superfood that helps prevent the common cold.

NOTE: Remember, elder is a tree with bark and not a small plant. There are some tall, poisonous hedgerow plants which also have sprays of white flowers – don't get confused with these – you don't want to make yourself a hemlock cordial!

Elderflower recipes

You can make some truly magical dishes with elderflowers! But first a few words of advice. Remember that all parts of the elder except from the flower and the cooked berry are slightly toxic. For this reason, I really recommend avoiding recipes where the whole flower head is thrown in; instead snip off the flowers with a pair of scissors.

I've also seen lots of recipes that call for washing the flower heads. This is a big no in my book! All the good stuff like the sweet pollen and wild yeast that will make your foods sing of sunshine sits on top of the flowers and is easily washed away (which is why you should never harvest elderflowers after a heavy rain). If you are worried about bugs, simply lay your elderflowers out on some paper and let them sit out for around half an hour so the bugs can scarper.

'You can make some truly magical dishes with elderflowers!'

Plant lore, folk medicine & magic

I feel I could write a whole book solely on the folklore around elder. It's so plentiful and so rich with symbolism, mystery, dark and light that it's easy to wonder if all the stories are about the same plant.

It has a very two-sided history: sometimes it's represented as a very sinister plant and sometimes as a generous and joyful one. *The Daily Chronicle* published an article in 1904 which read: 'It is popular superstition that a wound from an elder will prove fatal', which highlights its ominous reputation as a plant that causes harm and brings ill-fate. Similarly, to burn elder wood was thought to bring death and disaster and these negative connotations associated with the elder seem to have been so strong they still haven't disappeared completely.

In English and Scandinavian folklore, the elder was also known to be the home of the Elder Mother, a wise old goddess known to protect the elder and the wider woodland. A tale from Northamptonshire tells of man who cut a stick from an elder, and saw that the tree was bleeding. Later he meets the local witch and sees that she has a bloodied bandage on her arm. Witches are linked to the elder in many other ways too; in Ireland, witches rode eldersticks not broomsticks. It is still traditional to ask the Elder Mother before you take any of her offerings.

On the other hand, in Denmark, an elder twig put in the mouth was traditionally thought to drive out evil spirits and thus could cure toothache. In England, it was thought that the elder tree could never be hit by lightning and that carrying the twigs of an elder could protect their bearer from rheumatism. In some Slavic countries, such as Russia, it was thought that the tree had the power to ward off evil.

Elderflower cordial

This recipe is so simple and you can substitute elderflower for any sweet and fragrant wildflower. Once you have your cordial, mix it up with sparkling water for a fizzy treat, stir it up with icing sugar to drizzle over cakes or pour a little into a classic sponge cake mix.

**MAKES APPROX.
1 LITRE (4 CUPS)**

900g (4½ cups)
    granulated sugar
1.7 litres (7 cups)
    boiling water
3 unwaxed lemons
2 unwaxed oranges
30 elderflower
    heads
50g (2oz) citric acid
    (optional; you can
    buy this from the
    chemist or online)

1. Put the sugar into a large pan and add the boiling water. Stir until the sugar has dissolved.
2. Add the juice of 1 of the lemons and 1 of the oranges to the water. Slice the remaining lemons and oranges and add them to the water too.
3. Snip the flowers off the end of the elderflower heads over the pan, so they fall in too. Give everything a good stir and add the citric acid, if using (see Note). Cover the pan with a lid and leave to infuse for a minimum of 24 hours and up to 48 hours.
4. When your cordial has finished infusing, strain through a muslin cloth. It's best to do this over a large bowl first and then transfer to a lipped jug to pour into sterilised bottles.
5. This is ready to use straight away but will keep in the fridge for 1–6 weeks (see below). You can also freeze it if you'd like to preserve it for longer!

NOTE

The citric acid works to preserve the elderflower.
If it's been used, your cordial will keep in the fridge for up to 6 weeks. If you leave it out the cordial will last for about 1 week in the fridge before it starts to ferment.

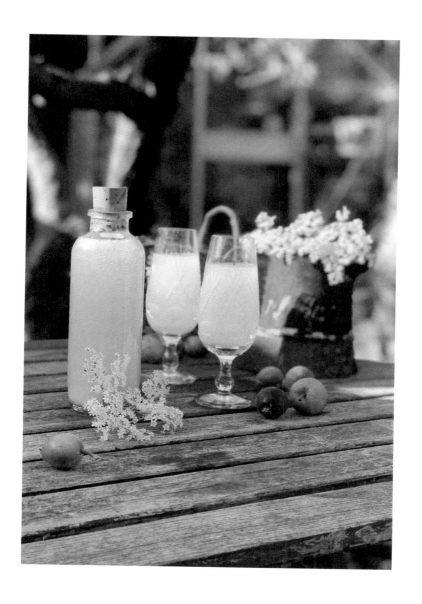

Elderflower Turkish delight

I first tried elderflower Turkish delight after reading the lovely John Wright's recipe and haven't stopped making it since. My recipe is made in the traditional way, so doesn't include any gelatine. It's soft, squishy and delightfully summery! Once you've got the hang of it, why not try this recipe with lilacs or lavender flowers instead?

**MAKES APPROX.
40 PIECES**

20 elderflower heads
4 tbsp lemon juice
750g (3¾ cups)
   white sugar
100g (¾ cup)
   cornflour
   (cornstarch) plus
   2 tbsp, for dusting
Coconut oil, for
   greasing
2 tbsp icing
   (confectioner's)
   sugar, for dusting

1. First, snip the flowers from the elderflower sprays from their stalks and put the loose flowers into the centre of a clean muslin cloth. Gather the sides of the cloth and tie with food safe string, so the flowers are contained. Make sure you leave a long piece of fabric or string to hold them while they're suspended in the pan. Put to the side for later.

2. In a large pan put 300ml water, the lemon juice and white sugar and heat gently and stir until the sugar has dissolved. Place a thermometer into the pan and bring the syrup to 250°F/120°C. This should take 15 – 30 minutes depending on your hob.

3. In a slightly smaller pan, mix the cornflour with 100ml water and mix until smooth. Now, over a low heat, add your cornflour mixture to the lemon syrup little by little, mixing all the time until combined.

4. Bring the mixture very slowly to the boil (slow simmering is key here, so use the smallest ring on your hob) and simmer for 10 minutes. Make sure you stir constantly. Now suspend the muslin bag with the flowers in the liquid and continue to simmer on a very low heat for another 20 minutes. Squeeze the bag with the back of your spoon to impart the most elderflower flavour possible.

5. The mixture will become very thick and almost clear. You will know it's ready when you can run your spoon through it, and the line drawn through the mixture holds its shape. When it's done, leave to cool slightly, for 10 minutes.

6. Line a square/rectangular cake tin with cling film and rub a little melted coconut oil over the film. Now pour in your Turkish delight mixture and leave to set overnight. In the morning put it in the fridge for a few hours before you cut it. When you're ready, cover a chopping board with the two tablespoons of cornflour mixed with the icing sugar. Turn out your Turkish delight on to the powdered board, cut into cubes and roll in the powder. The Turkish delight will last up to a month in an airtight container.

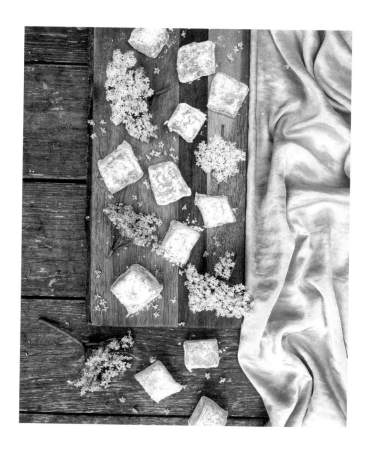

Wild Damson

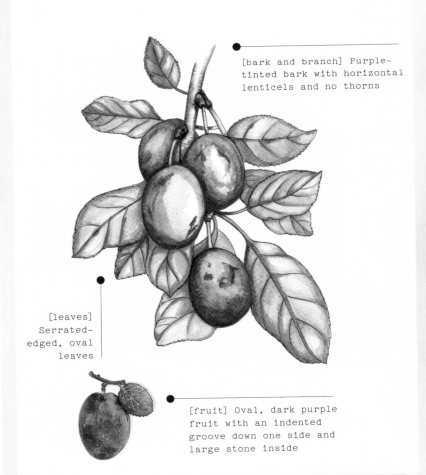

[bark and branch] Purple-tinted bark with horizontal lenticels and no thorns

[leaves] Serrated-edged, oval leaves

[fruit] Oval, dark purple fruit with an indented groove down one side and large stone inside

Foraging notes

Damsons are one of the most exciting gifts of summer. Reaching up to pluck a deep purple globe from a tree on a sun-dappled day and biting through the tart and slightly sour skin that bursts open with juice that runs down the chin never fails to bring a smile to my face.

Damsons, along with bullaces and greengages, are wild plums and for foraging purposes these can all be thought of as the same fruit, as they have very similar tastes and culinary uses. (You might also find cherry plums on your adventures, which are used in a slightly different way.)

Damsons are larger and sweeter than sloes and smaller and slightly more sour than shop-bought plums. They're ovaloid in shape and have a dark purple, dusty skin, which is tart to the taste with a soft fruity inside.

You might find a damson tree nestled among other trees in the hedgerows, on the outskirts of areas of wasteland or on the very edges of woodland. When you find your damson tree, take note of its location and return with a basket (and maybe even a stepladder if you're feeling committed!) when the fruits are ripening.

NOTE: There are many subspecies of plums, and you might even come across hybridised species. Many a pointless hour could be spent on arguing exactly which subspecies you've found, but I urge you to save your time and spend it in the happier pursuit of gathering and making damson treats to share with loved ones!

Damson recipes

I could eat a basket full of juicy, sweet damsons, without any fancy kitchen witchery any day of the week. Simply cut in half and twisted away from the pit is good enough for me. But they also make a wonderful addition to soft little vanilla cakes; dropping little slices of damson into your batter will leave you with gooey little pockets of fruitiness in your bake! They also make wonderful chutneys to enjoy with cheese, sweet sticky jams for toast, crumbles, pies and even boozy infusions!

Plant lore, folk medicine & magic

Damsons are packed with antioxidants, which protect your cells from damage by free radicals. The antioxidant polyphenol, which strengthens bones and helps reduce the risk of heart disease and diabetes, is very highly concentrated in damsons.

In Chinese mythology, the gods would feed plums to their favourite mortals to increase their vitality and strength, while in Japan, plums are often planted in the garden to protect against evil spirits.

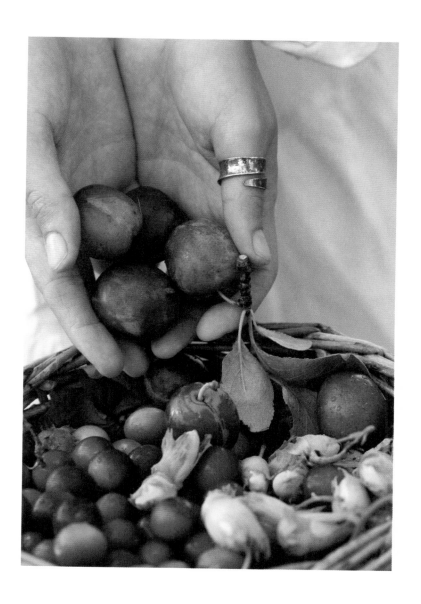

Plum galettes

These little fruit pies are incredibly easy to make and the perfect way to serve up a glut of wild fruits. Damsons work perfectly and look beautiful in their concentric circles, but you could also use blackberries, bilberries, cherries or apples. Best served warm with a scoop of ice cream!

MAKES 10

400g (14oz)
    large damsons
Small handful
    of blackberries
    (optional)
1 tbsp ground
    cinnamon
1 tbsp cornflour
    (cornstarch)
2 tbsp granulated
    sugar
1 tsp lemon juice
Milk or beaten egg,
    for brushing
Flaked almonds or
    granulated sugar,
    to top

For the pastry
300g (2¼ cups)
    plain (all-purpose)
    flour, plus extra
    for dusting
½ tsp salt
150g (5oz) butter,
    chilled and diced
2 tbsp icing
    (confectioner's)
    sugar
3 tbsp ice-cold water

1. First make the pastry. Before you start, make sure your ingredients and equipment are fridge cold, including your mixing bowl. Put the flour, salt and butter into a food processor and pulse briefly until the mixture resembles breadcrumbs. Tip into your bowl, then stir in the icing sugar.

2. Make a well in the centre of the bowl and gradually pour in the cold water. Use your hands to bring the mixture together into a dough (avoid overworking too much). Form into a ball and wrap in cling film and leave in the fridge for at least 30 minutes (or overnight if you want to make this in advance).

3. While your pastry is chilling, prepare the filling: de-stone the damsons and thinly slice them. Pop them into a bowl with the whole blackberries, if using. Add the cinnamon, cornflour, sugar and lemon juice and stir until the fruit is evenly coated.

4. Divide the pastry into two and leave one half in the fridge. Allow the second half to sit for 10 minutes at room temperature before rolling it out on a floured surface to the thickness of a pound coin.

5. Cut around a medium bowl to create three circles of pastry, then collect up the leftover pastry, reroll and repeat to cut another two circles. Repeat with the second half of the pastry.

6. Arrange the circles of pastry on two baking sheets. Place the slices of damson in circles in the centre of the pastry and pop some blackberries in the centre.

7. Fold the edges of each galette over to tuck in the fruit, leaving a circle of exposed fruit in the middle. Crimp the pastry to keep the whole thing compact.
8. Brush the edges of the pastry with milk or beaten egg and sprinkle over the flaked almonds or granulated sugar, then chill the galettes in the fridge for a few hours. I sometimes sprinkle mine with a few hogweed seeds.
9. Preheat the oven to 190°C/375°F/gas 5 and bake the galettes for 25 minutes, or until the pastry is golden brown and the fruit is bubbling.

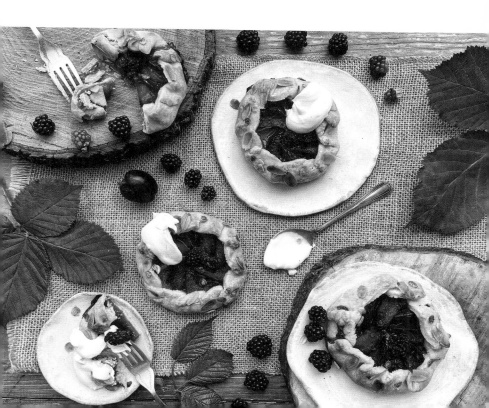

Charred damson salad

This is our go-to savoury recipe for damsons. Charring the plums brings out their natural jammy sweetness, which goes so incredibly well with a rich, creamy cheese, a sharp balsamic glaze and a peppery salad leaf.

SERVES 2 AS A MAIN OR 4 AS A SIDE

60g (2oz) butter
1 tbsp olive oil
8–10 damsons, halved and pitted
Bag of mixed summer salad leaves (nasturtium, rocket and watercress work well)
250g (9oz) fresh goat's cheese
A handful of toasted walnuts or pumpkin seeds
Olive oil and elderberry balsamic glaze (see page 233), for drizzling
Sea salt and freshly ground black pepper

1. Heat the butter and oil in a frying pan over a high heat. Arrange the damsons in the pan, cut side down, and cook until the plums are slightly blackened, about 5 minutes. Transfer to a plate and leave to cool slightly, cut side up.

2. Assemble the salad by placing the leaves in a serving bowl, then top with the plums. Crumble the cheese over and sprinkle over the nuts or seeds.

3. Dress generously with olive oil and balsamic glaze and season with salt and pepper. Serve immediately.

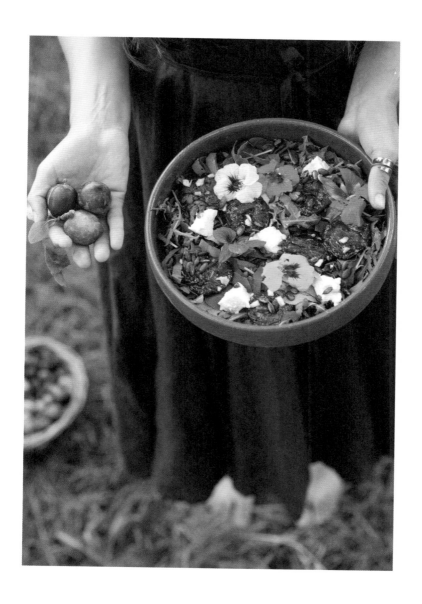

Mugwort

[buds] Silvery
buds with a
sage-like smell

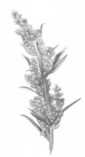

[structure]
Tall stands
of individual
red- to purple-
tinged stems

[leaves] Deeply
segregated and
usually in five
to seven lobes
with silvery
undersides

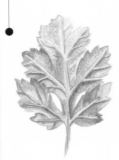

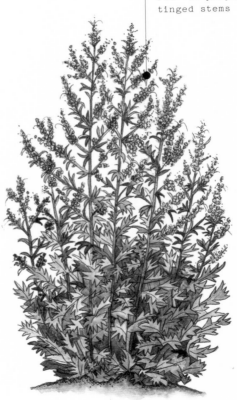

Foraging notes

Hot, dry days lead to flourishing stands of Mother Mugwort! A beautifully mellow and slightly bitter aromatic herb, it can be used in so many recipes and rituals. It's a particularly ancient herb and can be dated as far back as 2,000 years ago, featuring in some Chinese poems and songs.

Mugwort is usually found by the edge of the road or lining the footpaths and rarely in the middle of meadows. Once it goes to flower, producing tall spikes of silvery green buds, it's easy to see from far away. To harvest, simply take a few leaves or a handful of flowering stems.

When crushed the leaves have a herby sage- or lavender-like smell. Mugwort is most traditionally used for flavouring beer but has also been used as a spice, as food, as medicine, as a spiritual aid, in acupuncture (moxibustion is the traditional Chinese practice of burning mugwort leaves to promote healing with acupuncture) and as a moth and insect repellent in the garden.

NOTE: This herb isn't recommended for anyone who is pregnant or breastfeeding.

Mugwort recipes

Mugwort leaves and buds can both be used for food in a similar way to sage. I love to throw some mugwort sprigs in with a tin of roasting veg, and even to throw some sprigs into a warming hot chocolate for those cooler summer nights.

For rituals and self-care, I love to use mugwort for its relaxing and cleansing qualities, either as a simple smoke stick to burn and create a meditative atmosphere or in a soothing foot bath after a long day of hiking.

Plant lore, folk medicine & magic

Mugwort is fantastic at relaxing the muscles! St John the Baptist was said to line his sandals with it, so when he walked to spread the word of God, his foot would crush the herb and release relaxing essential oils into the sole of the foot. It works wonderfully on an internal level too; I always have a mugwort tea when I've got my period as it is said to stimulate menstruation and can ease cramps (for this reason it's probably best to avoid it if you are pregnant or breastfeeding).

Mugwort was one of the Saxons' six sacred herbs and they believed it was given to mortals by the god Woden. They used to smoke it as incense to cleanse areas or people and drive away evil spirits! It's also long been used for its psychic and prophetic properties. It is a very mild psychoactive plant and can induce very vivid and even lucid dreams. The Saxons believed these dreams were prophetic and important messages could be found within them.

Mugwort hot chocolate

Mugwort's earthy, dreamy, sage-like flavours complement a warming cup of rich hot chocolate amazingly. As a powerful relaxant with the ability to help you venture into a world of lucid dreaming, it adds a whole handful of magic to your bedtime drink! Make it over a fire in the woods as the summer sun sets and drink as you imagine your body rooting down into the earth and your spirit soaring.

SERVES 2

600ml (2½ cups) milk of your choice
60g (2oz) dark chocolate (at least 70% cocoa solids)
2–3 sprigs of mugwort buds
½ tsp vanilla bean paste

1. Add the milk to a small saucepan and heat gently until steaming.
2. Grate or finely chop the dark chocolate and add it into the pan. Continue to heat the milk for a few moments while stirring, until the chocolate melts.
3. Add the mugwort sprigs and allow to steep for 2-3 minutes or until the hot chocolate is fragrant with the scent of mugwort.
4. Take off the heat, stir in the vanilla paste and pour into mugs.

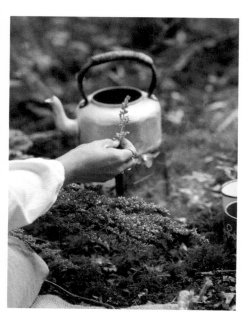

Mugwort mochi

Some parts of Japan and Korea use mugwort in a similar way to matcha. It's either puréed or powdered and used to flavour lattes, cakes, ice creams and … mochi! Mochi are soft, chewy little puddings made from glutinous rice flour. They usually take a lot of work, but this cheat's recipe makes them super-easy!

MAKES 6

Handful of fresh mugwort leaves
200ml (generous ¾ cup) boiling water
Small handful of dried mugwort leaves (optional)
70g (2½oz) glutinous rice flour
15g (½oz) granulated sugar
30g (⅓ cup) cornflour (cornstarch), for dusting
6 scoops of vanilla ice cream, about 30g (2oz) each, individually portioned out and frozen

1. First make your mugwort tea: put the mugwort leaves (and some of the buds if they are available) into a jug or teapot and pour over the boiling water. Cover and leave to steep for at least 5 minutes, or until it tastes strong but not bitter. Measure out 100ml (3½fl oz) of the tea to use in this recipe.
2. Now make you mugwort powder (this step is optional, but I recommend as it will give your motchi extra mugwort flavour). Grind or process your dried mugwort leaves in a spice grinder or a pestle and mortar until very fine. If using a pestle and mortar you may also want to sieve the ground leaves to create a finer powder. Measure out 10g (¼oz) of this powder.
3. Now for the dough. Put the glutinous rice flour, mugwort powder, mugwort tea and sugar into a shallow bowl and stir to combine. Cover the bowl and microwave for 2–3 minutes, stopping at 1-minute intervals to stir the mixture. It will thicken and become translucent.
4. Divide the dough into six equal portions and roll each into a ball. Use a rolling pin dusted with cornflour to roll out and flatten into a round circles. Let the dough cool a little bit.
5. Place a frozen ball of ice cream in the centre of each circle of dough, then quickly pinch the seams together. Remember to work quickly so the ice cream doesn't melt.
6. Dust each ball with additional cornflour and return to the freezer until solid, about 4–6 hours.
7. Remove the mochi balls from the freezer about 5–10 minutes before serving.

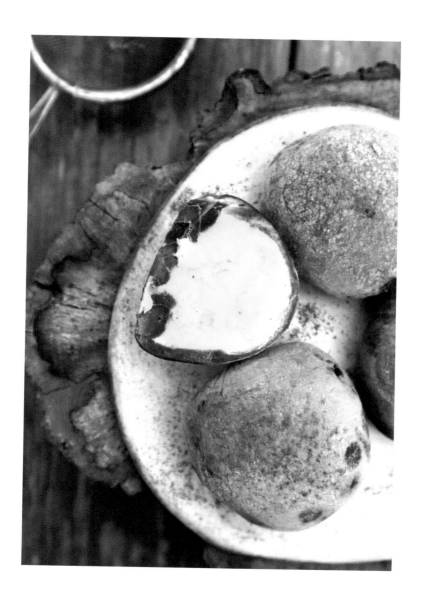

Pineapple Weed

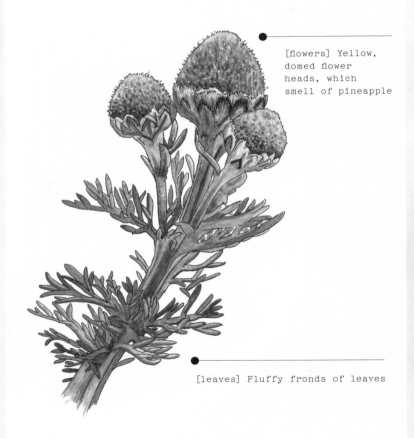

[flowers] Yellow, domed flower heads, which smell of pineapple

[leaves] Fluffy fronds of leaves

Foraging notes

Someone once described pineapple weed to me as a bald chamomile, which I thought was perfect. It looks incredibly similar to chamomile, but has no white petals round the flower heads. When crushed between the fingers, pineapple weed flower heads smell exactly like pineapple gummy sweets. It's the most delightfully surprising smell to come across in a British hedgerow and that flavour can be lent (when used in the right way) to many sweet dishes and sweets!

Lots of people will search high and low for this plant, scouring their wild spaces and the corners of little-trodden fields, when in fact it's much more likely to be found in the car park, or in the cracks between the pavements. It loves poor soil and heavily trampled areas.

Pineapple weed recipes

There are so many ways to use pineapple weed heads. Chop up and stir into cookies or cake mixes, infuse with cream overnight and then whip the cream for a delicious filling for eclairs, or maybe you'd like to make a boozy alcohol infusion?

Don't forget that the leaves of pineapple weed are edible too. Use them in herbal teas for their relaxing, sleep-inducing qualities, or throw a handful into a salad.

One thing to note, you might want to give them a little rinse before using! I don't say that much, but it's very hard to find pineapple weed growing off the beaten track.

Plant lore, folk medicine & magic

Pineapple weed was used plentifully for its medicinal and magical properties by multiple Native American tribes. Medicinally it was used to relax the nervous system and ease digestive cramps, among other things.

This plant was also reportedly used as part of the Northern Cheyenne Sun Dance. The dance was performed at important ceremonies to renew the people and the earth. A herbal mixture containing the tops of pineapple weed would be chewed up and blown on the participants for its cooling effect.

It's also believed to have been burned with human hair to prevent a loved one from leaving. Similarly it was thought to prevent a horse from running away when it was burned with horse hair.

Pineapple weed shortbread

These little biscuits are buttery, crumbly and delicate with a soft and fruity flavour of pineapple weed. They bring joy and relaxation to any mid-day herbal tea break and make wonderful gifts.

You can roll these biscuits out to any shape. I like to roll them thin so they melt in the mouth, but a more rustic approach is always fun too. To do this, press the dough into a 8-inch cake tin, bake the whole thing and then cut into chunky slices like my Nan used to do! (Add around 25 minutes to your cook time for this option.)

MAKES 20 BISCUITS

200g (7oz) soft butter (good-quality, solid butter, not marge, if you're choosing plant-based)
100g (½ cup) caster sugar
½ tsp vanilla extract
1 tsp salt
300g (1¾ cups) plain flour, plus extra for dusting
2 tbsp chopped fresh pineapple weed heads
1 tbsp granulated sugar for topping (optional)

1. Preheat the oven to 160°C and line two baking trays with parchment paper.
2. Let the butter sit out of the fridge for at least one hour to soften.
3. In a bowl, cream the soft butter, sugar, vanilla and salt together until smooth and creamy.
4. In a separate bowl, sift the flour and stir through the pineapple weed flower heads until evenly distributed.
5. Stir the flour into the butter and sugar until a crumbly dough has formed. Wrap this in a waxed cloth or cling film and chill in the fridge for at least 30 minutes.
6. Remove the dough from the fridge, place on a floured surface and roll out to around ½cm in thickness.
7. Use a biscuit cutter to cut out rounds and place them on your baking tray. Sprinkle each biscuit with a little granulated sugar.
8. Cook for 12-15 minutes or until very lightly golden. Remove from the oven and allow to cool.

Pineapple weed mojito

This wild cocktail is epic and a summer favourite in my house! A whole level up from your average mojito, you'll get a tropical, pineappley flavour from the pineapple weed and a deep, minty, herbal flavour from the ground ivy.

MAKES 1 TALL GLASS

For the pineapple weed-infused rum
Handful of pineapple weed flower heads
125ml (½ cup) good-quality white rum

For the pineapple weed mojito
1 tbsp soft light brown sugar
Juice of 1 lime
Small handful of ground ivy (see page 72)
90ml (3fl oz) pineapple weed-infused rum
Ice cubes
Tonic water or soda water, to top
Ground ivy leaves and edible flowers, to decorate

1. To make the pineapple weed-infused rum, add your pineapple weed heads and rum to a clean jam jar with a tight-fitting lid and leave for 3–5 days until the pineapple flavour has infused the rum. Shaking the jar daily will help infuse the flavour.

2. When your pineapple weed rum has infused, strain out the pineapple weed heads. If they're left in the rum too long, it will become bitter and overpowering.

3. To make your mojito, put the sugar, lime juice and ground ivy into a tall glass or jar. Muddle (you can use the end of a wooden spoon or a pestle if you don't have a cocktail muddler) to crush the herbs and release the flavour.

4. Add the pineapple weed-infused rum, fill the glass with ice and stir.

5. Top up with tonic or soda water and stir again.

6. Decorate your glass and enjoy!

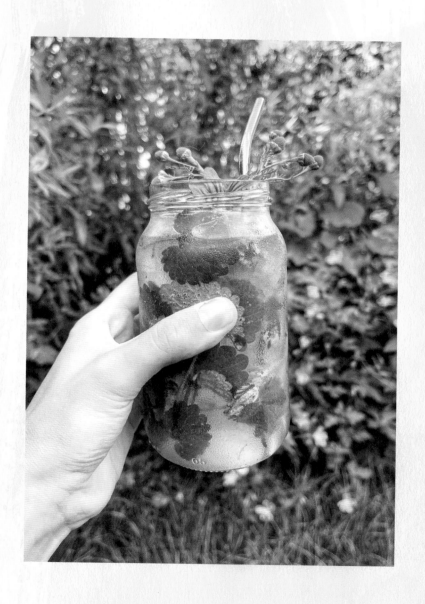

Yarrow

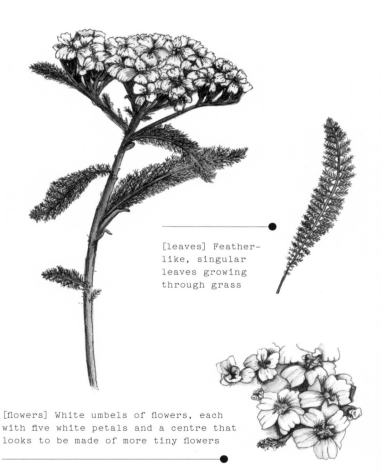

[leaves] Feather-
like, singular
leaves growing
through grass

[flowers] White umbels of flowers, each
with five white petals and a centre that
looks to be made of more tiny flowers

Foraging notes

Yarrow is an ancient healing herb, with a huge array of medicinal uses and some delicious edible ones too! You'll find yarrow growing in meadows, lawns and fields, among the grass. When it comes into flower in summer, the white flower heads will help you find the young, feather-like, fluffy green leaves.

Yarrow is also known as soldier's woundwort, staunch weed and knight's milfoil, which helpfully points towards its most common, or most highly valued, use throughout history: staunching blood (see page 154).

NOTE: This herb isn't recommended for anyone who is pregnant or breastfeeding.

Yarrow recipes

When using yarrow in the kitchen, you want to pick the tender young leaves. You'll notice that young yarrow leaves are soft to the touch and bright green. As they get older they become darker green and tough. The young leaves lend flavours of parsley and mild dill to savoury dishes and can be used in the same way. Try making yarrow leaf tempura or throwing a handful of yarrow into a fresh salad or pesto. The flowers can also be used for infusions, tea and tinctures. If yarrow is out of season, or you're having trouble finding it, you can still make these recipes by substituting in fresh dill.

Plant lore, folk medicine & magic

The Greek hero Achilles was told by his mentor Chiron, the centaur, that with the use of yarrow, he could heal his army's wounds after every battle and go on to win another.

I am lucky enough to have experienced the traditional application of yarrow for its wound-staunching abilities first hand. In 2019 my soul sister Ruby and I were travelling in the Philippines and were staying on a remote island. She'd gone to do some yoga in the woods and fell onto a branch, which lodged itself in the very fleshy bit of her upper thigh. She came back to the hostel with blood pouring down her leg. In England, it would have been a trip to A&E and a few stitches but the Filipina woman who ran the hostel told her to sit down and apply pressure while she went to get something. Ruby was confident this 'something' would be a doctor. But it turned out to be a fistful of yarrow.

The woman cleaned up the wound and then mashed up the herbs in a pestle and mortar and packed the open wound, pushing the herbs into the hole and then wrapping it with bandages. The woman continued to change the herbs three times a day. We were astounded at how quickly the wound was healing. Ruby said it felt very different to modern medicine too, almost as if she could feel her body responding to the herbs, rather than feeling like something was being done to her.

It was an amazing experience (perhaps more for me than for Ruby!) to be able to see how yarrow would have been used to treat wounds before modern medicine. And what made it even more special was to know that there are still some places in the world where herbs are still valued and utilised for their incredible healing benefits.

Creamy yarrow dip

A dollop of this creamy, herby dip is delicious on most dishes, from lasagne to homemade baked beans. But it's also perfect to dunk your crisps, roast potatoes or carrot and cucumber sticks into.

SERVES 4 GENEROUSLY

240g (1 cup) sour cream
80ml (⅓ cup) mayonnaise
1 tbsp onion powder
1 tbsp garlic powder
1 tbsp dried yarrow (or 2 tbsp finely chopped fresh yarrow)
1 tsp salt
Finely chopped fresh yarrow, to garnish

1. Place all the ingredients into a bowl and stir until combined. Taste and adjust the seasoning if necessary.
2. Sprinkle over the fresh yarrow and serve.

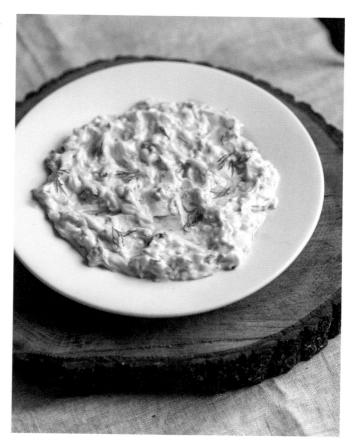

Yarrow and lemon potatoes

Yarrow goes very well with potatoes, whether it's in a light, summery potato salad, layered in a creamy potato dauphinoise or my personal favourite, baked with a tray of roasties, perfect for dipping in some creamy yarrow dip (see page 155) or maybe some hawthorn ketchup (see page 210).

SERVES 4

700g (1½lb) good roasting potatoes (e.g. Maris Piper)
3 tbsp olive oil
2 garlic cloves, finely chopped or grated
1 tsp dried yarrow
Juice of ½ lemon
1 tbsp finely chopped fresh yarrow
Sea salt and freshly ground black pepper

1. Preheat the oven to 230°C/450°F/gas 8.
2. Chop the potatoes into even-sized chunks or wedges and put into a baking tray. Your potatoes should be in one layer and have a little space around each one for maximum crispiness.
3. Drizzle over the olive oil and scatter over the garlic along with the dried yarrow and salt and pepper. Toss well to combine, so each potato is coated in oil.
4. Bake your potatoes for 20 minutes, turning halfway through. They're ready when they're crispy on the outside and soft in the middle (you can test this with a fork).
5. Remove from the oven, squeeze over the lemon juice and stir through the finely chopped fresh yarrow.
6. Serve immediately as a side dish or with a dip of your choice!

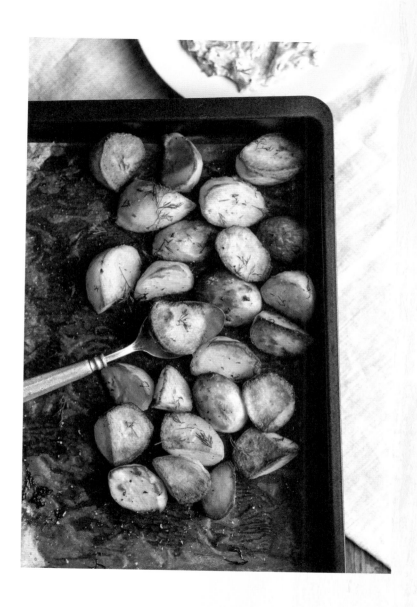

Summer Self-care

While summer is a glorious time to celebrate and socialise, it's also the perfect season to take some time for stillness, reflection and self-care.

Sometimes the rush of summer can feel overwhelming and everything and everyone seems to speed up. The world around us becomes a hive of activity and we inevitably get less sleep. The hot sun and salty swims can take their toll and leave us feeling not so fresh too. But with a few simple summer rituals, you can balance out these effects and welcome in the summer while nourishing your body and soul.

Take some time to sit and meditate frequently and consider the light and dark energies in your life. Forage slowly and mindfully for herbs that call out to you and will help ease any imbalances. Brew yourself a herbal tea or take some time to pamper your skin and welcome in the slowness that comes alongside these activities.

'Welcome in the summer
while nourishing your body
and soul.'

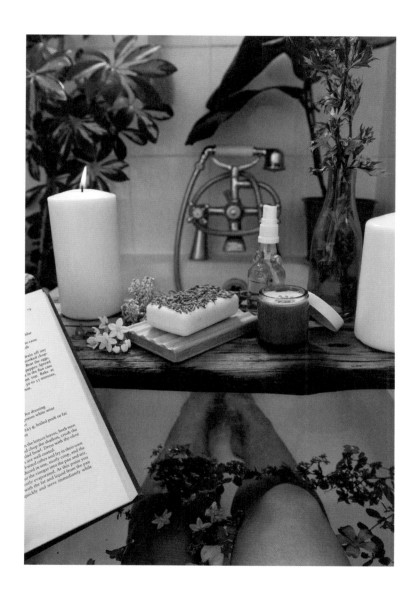

Summer Rituals

Make a wild herbal tea

Making a wild herbal tea can be so much more than popping the kettle on and hurriedly sipping between everyday jobs. Done right, it can be a personal journey and beneficial ritual which will help you to harmonise with nature, engage your senses and balance your energetic levels.

When you go out to pick your herbs, try to choose the edible herbs or flowers that call out to you and pick them mindfully and intentionally. Feel them between your fingertips, thank them for their offering.

Now it's time to make your tea, which you can do at home, or out in nature, over a little burner. You'll need roughly ¼ cup of fresh herbs (or ⅛ cup of dried herbs) per cup of water. Boil your water, turn off the heat and then add your herbs and allow them to steep, covered, for 3–4 minutes, or until you're happy with the strength of your tea.

If you don't have time for this ritual in its entirety, or if you're simply making a quick batch of tea for a recipe, you can of course use wild dried herbs from your larder and enjoy an abridged version at home.

HERBS FOR TEA

Yarrow for …
hormone regulation. To protect from negative energy and heal emotional wounds.

Mugwort for …
its muscle-relaxing qualities. To enhance lucid dreams and enhance psychic powers.

Pineapple weed for …
its calming and cleansing qualities. To welcome in resilience and joy.

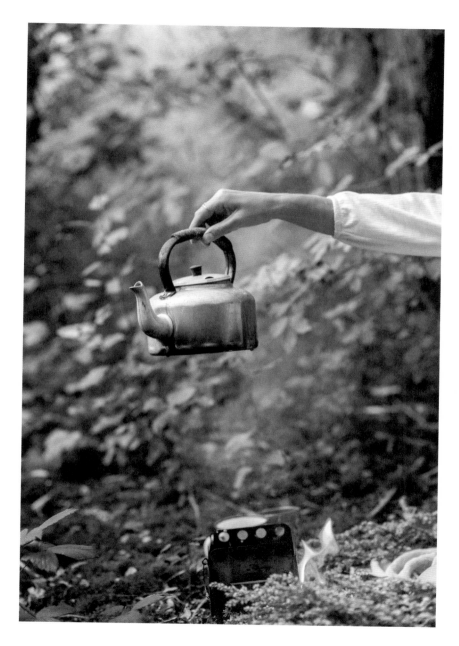

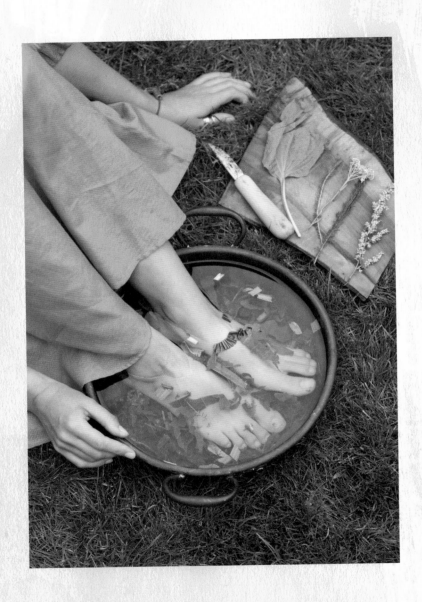

Celebrate the summer solstice

The summer solstice is the longest day of the year, usually falling on 21 June. It's the day the sun reaches its highest point in the sky and marks midsummer.

We know that midsummer celebrations or rituals have been held across almost all cultures in the northern hemisphere, as far back as the Neolithic era, when ancient people erected stone circles to line up with the movement of the sun on this sacred day.

Why was such emphasis placed on this day? The answer is we don't really know, but we can be pretty certain that for hunter-gatherers, people so reliant on the cycles of nature, the longest day of the year would have held huge significance. The sun brought warmth, allowed crops to grow and signalled the start and end of each day. What better time to celebrate its magic, than on the day when it reaches its highest point in the sky?

Why not hold your own celebration of the summer solstice – whether it's by simply making the most of those few extra minutes of sunlight and watching the sun go down, or go all the way and light a bonfire to dance naked around? For me, it always has to be a picnic – simple as that. I love to get out of the midday sun, shelter under a shady tree and enjoy some wild foods to remind me of the power of the sun.

Make a herbal footbath

A long summer of foraging, hiking and hobbling across stony beaches to the sea will leave your feet in need of some love! Footbaths have been shown to improve circulation in the feet, reduce stress and even improve sleep.

The soles of the feet are incredibly absorbent and will soak up all the lovely essential oils from your wild herbs, making the most of their wonderfully medicinal qualities.

To make a herbal footbath, gather a few handfuls of wild herbs and roughly shred. Put the herbs into a large flat-bottomed container and pour over boiling water until the container is around a third full. Allow your herbs to steep for 10 minutes and then top up with cold water until your footbath is the desired temperature. Pop your feet in, sit back and enjoy!

Try rose and lavender for a relaxing footbath, plantain, yarrow and mugwort for a healing footbath, or if it's a sunny day, add lots of cool water and use refreshing, anti-inflammatory herbs like mint and nettle.

Burn smoke sticks for a magical midsummer cleanse

Mysticism and magic have been at the heart of summer solstice folklore in cultures across the world. Magic was thought to be strongest during the summer solstice and myths told stories of the world turning upside down or the sun standing still at midsummer.

Summer solstice is the perfect time of year for a ritual. Try burning wild, dried herbs to help you put any trials from the first half of the year behind you, welcome in energies for the second half and ask the universe for something that seems out of reach. Instead of the more well-known white sage, try creating smoke sticks with bundles of dried mugwort, lavender and rosemary to burn as a midsummer cleansing ritual.

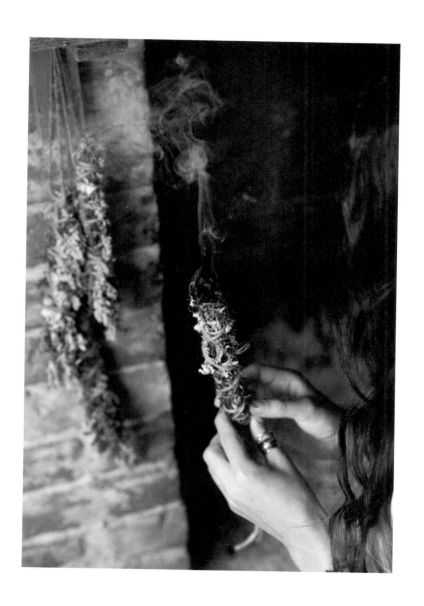

Autumn

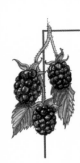

After a long dazzling summer, September rolls in like a cool breeze. It brings with it the promise of ripening hedgerow fruits, forest floors littered with hazel shells and, later, abundant displays of fungi of all varieties. Squirrels and dormice are about to begin the busy hunt to stock their winter larders and it's time for us to do the same!

Autumn arrives with a glut of hedgerow fruits and nuts, branches heavy with apples, thorny bushes filled with ruby-red hawthorns and tender green hazels growing stronger in the sun. Full baskets transform into fruit roll ups and warming fruit pies with generous pinches of mixed spice and cinnamon.

The leaves start to turn golden brown and drift gently to the ground as the temperatures drop and the nights get longer. A breath of calm settles over the land and the urge to hold hot drinks in cold hands and snuggle under blankets takes over.

As we move into the second half of autumn, there seems to be something magical in the air. The sun glitters through the trees in the woodland on chilly days and your breath suddenly becomes visible. A haze of smoke, a word transformed – for only a moment – into a being, floating on the air.

In October the rains come, and the fallen leaves turn into a glorious brown pulp, which is slowly consumed by mycelial networks. The little white fibres that make up these networks slowly creep through the earth, turning dying matter into rich soil, eventually fruiting beautiful, ethereal mushrooms. Of all colours and sizes, they appear – a mysterious wonder to behold and, if you're lucky, a prize edible to enjoy!

Autumn is a time to relax into the slowness of the coming months and to revel in cosiness and contentment.

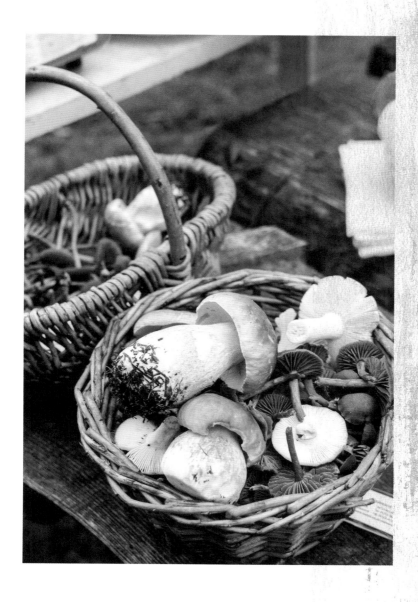

Foraging in Autumn

In the autumn, hedgerow fruits ripen, thickets of bramble become heavy with their autumn offerings, and blackberries wait to be turned into jams, pies and blackberry wine. Tall rowan trees present droops of sour orange berries on graceful limbs, the perfect ingredient for a wild alternative to cranberry sauce. The Elder Mother prepares to guide us into the darker months, sharing her sprays of tiny black elderberries, with the most powerful immune-supporting qualities.

It's not just hedgerow fruits but also nuts, wild seeds and spices that we can harvest throughout early autumn. Protein-packed wild beech nuts and hazelnuts can be eaten fresh or blended into nut butter or even made into wild 'Nutella'!

Mushrooms

There is something distinctly magical about foraging for mushrooms. The herbs, berries and nuts that we forage year after year become somewhat reliable and constant. If we move to a new area, we have plenty of clues to tell us where we might find our favourite ingredients. Want to harvest acorns in the autumn? Head to that park with all the oaks, of course. Mushrooms, on the other hand, remain much more of a mystery, most likely because the majority of the organism lives out of sight, under the ground.

Mycelium is the main organism that mushrooms grow from. If you've ever picked up a mound of earth and seen it marbled with a very fine white webbing, that's mycelium. This network of white fibres, or hyphae, feeds on and breaks down dead and decaying matter and is the reason we can take strolls through the woodland without having to wade through leaf litter and fallen branches. It's the greatest recycler we know, transforming dying matter into rich and nutritious soil.

When the web of mycelium runs out of nutrients it will send up a mushroom (under the right conditions) to spread spores. These spores are usually carried on the wind and will settle in the earth slightly further afield than the mushroom. Spores are like microscopic seeds and will grow into another mycelial network, which will eventually connect with the original network, providing more nutrients from dead or decaying matter.

Mycelial networks don't just pass nutrients throughout their systems but have the ability to send electrical signals too. And their communication doesn't stop at the fungal kingdom either; it's been proven that plants and trees use the mycelial networks to communicate and send nutrients between themselves too. It's one of the reasons they're sometimes called the 'wood-wide-web'.

To say that mushrooms are a complete mystery is not quite correct; they don't pop up entirely randomly. Specific mycelium prefers certain environments and will form connections to certain types of trees. One that network is established, it will fruit with mushrooms for at least several years.

Uncovering the mysteries surrounding mushrooms can not only lead to a delightfully delicious basketful of edible wild mushrooms, but also to some eye-opening knowledge about a completely unique and magical kingdom: the fungi kingdom. Mushrooms come in some weird and wonderful forms and the study of them, known as mycology, is an incredible thing; I've found myself foraging for facts just as joyfully as I forage for mushrooms!

When it comes to foraging for mushrooms, I know many would prefer it to be more straightforward. Mushrooms pop up for a few months of the year in the right weather conditions and according to the Woodland Trust there are over 15,000 species in the UK, some of them deadly. Mushroom foraging is a skill that you will develop over years, not weeks, but it's important to know is that there are plenty of common, beginner-friendly mushrooms with no toxic lookalikes. Here are some beginner-friendly shrooms to start you on your journey:

Puffballs
Giant puffballs
Penny buns

Chanterelles
Parasols
Field mushrooms

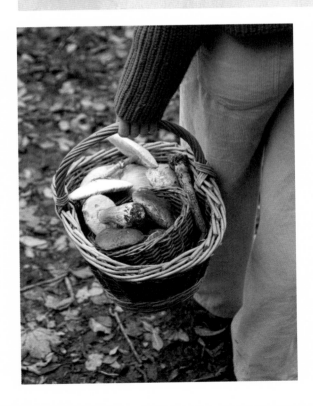

Nuts

There's a surprising number of nut-bearing trees out there in our woodlands and parks, ranging from the more well-known (walnut and hazel) to the lesser-known (oak, beech and sweet chestnut).

After foraging fresh nuts a few years in a row, you'll notice that the amount of nuts on offer can differ hugely. Some years will be very thin on the ground, but other years almost every oak, beech or chestnut in the country will provide an absolute abundance of nuts! These are known as mast years. How the trees co-ordinate themselves is a mystery yet to be uncovered but it's thought to be a method of ensuring enough nuts are left over for young saplings to grow!

When we're foraging, it's so important to always leave a good number of nuts for wildlife. Squirrels, mice and birds all rely on nuts to fatten up on over the winter. The good news is, in a good year, plenty of huge, meaty nuts can be harvested without making a dent in what's available for the wildlife.

Nuts would have been an incredibly important resource for hunter-gatherer humans. An archaeological dig in Israel found seven varieties of nuts, along with stone tools to crack them open, dating from around 780,000 years ago. (They were found deep in a bog and so were very well preserved.)

In general, nuts are a good source of fat, fibre and protein. Most of the fat in nuts is healthy monounsaturated fat (as opposed to the saturated fat we find in fast food), as well as omega 6 and omega 3 polyunsaturated fat. Nuts also pack a number of vitamins and minerals, including magnesium and vitamin E. They're also an incredibly versatile ingredient: they can be eaten fresh or roasted in a huge number of dishes, ground into flour or pressed into oil. Considering how expensive shop-bought nuts are, autumn is a brilliant time to get a good harvest of free, wild nuts.

Crab Apple

[leaves] Pointed
oval leaves with
serrated edges

[bark and branch]
Grey and scaly bark

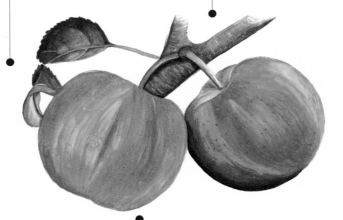

[fruit] Small apples 1—7cm (½—
2¾in) across; cut them in half
horizontally to see a seed star

Foraging notes

Nothing brings more joy to my heart than a heavily laden apple tree, whether it's the apple tree in my mum's garden or the crab apple tree on my favourite country walk. Crab apples are much smaller, slightly scabbier and much more sour than apples, but just as delightful!

Seeing those shining green and red globes is such a comfort and immediately awakens the senses with the memory of the smell of apple pie and the taste of tangy apple cider vinegar. Apples really do come in a spectrum of sweet to sour; biting into one will quickly tell you what you might want to do with it. Crab apples will often make the mouth water like sour sweets and should be cooked before they're eaten.

Apples have always symbolised abundance and when you're standing on a rickety stepladder plucking fruits from the branches and popping them into an already full basket, it's clear why! That basket will lend itself to so many meals, desserts, jams and chutneys – you could be enjoying those apples in some form for the whole year.

Crab apple recipes

Apples are a superb ingredient for making a huge range of sweet and savoury dishes. Here are just two of my favourites but remember it doesn't stop there! Try tarte tatin, apple crisps or – if you harvest a larger amount – how about making your own chutney, cider or apple cider vinegar?

You can use any type of crab apples for these recipes but remember to taste them first. If they are especially sour, you may want to increase the sugar in the following recipes. If you're using eating apples from your garden or a local orchard, you may want to reduce it.

Plant lore, folk medicine & magic

Apples have had huge spiritual significance in many cultures throughout history and the world over. They've long been connected to abundance and prosperity.

The ancient tradition of wassailing (see page 281), originating from pagan times, is one that is still performed and celebrated throughout England in January. Various ceremonies are performed in apple orchards to ensure an abundant harvest in the coming year. The ceremonies include banging pots, pans and drums to scare away evil spirits, hanging toast dipped in cider from the trees and singing to invite good spirits, and the passing round of a communal wassail bowl, filled with mulled cider for attendees.

The apple is also a favoured tool for divination, where the whole apple is peeled in one, the peel then tossed over the shoulder, where it lands and reveals the letter of the first name of the man or woman you will fall in love with.

'Apples have long been connected to abundance and prosperity.'

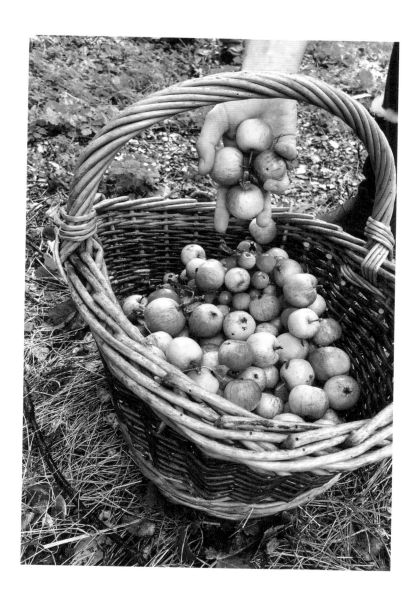

Toffee apple doughnuts

I'm not the biggest fan of toffee apples, but I love traditional foods that go with traditional celebrations! So, here's my spin on a toffee apple – soft, fluffy doughnuts filled with spiced apple sauce and drizzled with a toffee sauce made with a good pinch of smoked sea salt for a smoky bonfire night flavour.

MAKES 6

1½ tbsp ground flaxseed
100ml (3½fl oz) cold water
375g (3 cups) strong white bread flour, plus extra for dusting
300g (1½ cups) caster (superfine) sugar
10g (⅓oz) instant dried yeast
30g (1oz) dairy-free butter
7g (¼oz) superfine salt
145ml (⅔ cup) oat milk
60ml (¼ cup) warm water
1 litre (4 cups) vegetable oil, for frying

1. Make a flaxseed egg by combining the ground flaxseed and cold water in a small bowl. Leave for 20 minutes until it reaches a gelatinous consistency.
2. Place the flour, 40g (1½oz) of the sugar and the yeast in the bowl of a stand mixer and combine. Add the butter, salt, flaxseed egg and oat milk. Use the dough hook attachment and mix on a slow speed while slowly pouring in the warm water.
3. When the ingredients are combined and you have used all the water, continue to knead in the mixer on a slow setting for around 8 minutes until you have an elastic, smooth and shiny dough.
4. Put the dough in a lightly oiled bowl and cover with a waxed cloth or damp towel until doubled in sized.
5. Dust a work surface with flour and tip your dough out and pull the edges of the dough in to form a ball. Sprinkle a rolling pin with flour and roll the dough to around 2cm (¾in) thick.
6. Fill a small, heavy-based saucepan three-quarters full with vegetable oil and heat to 180°C (350°F), or until a small piece of dough rises to the surface and very gently bubbles around the edges. You may need to top up the oil in between each doughnut.
7. Use a round cutter to cut six doughnuts and leave to rise for 10 minutes, or until the dough bounces back when pressed.

Recipe continues over the page

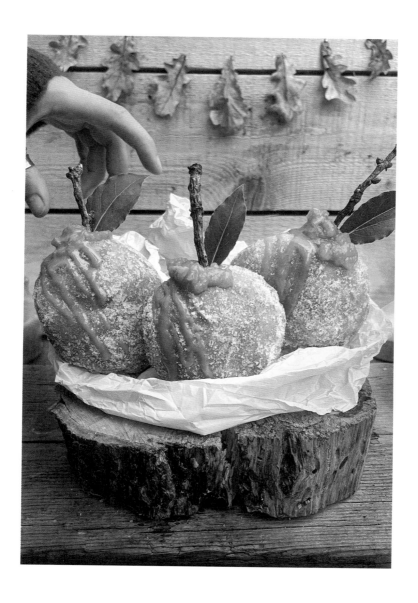

For the filling

400g (14oz) peeled, cored and cubed crab apples
65g (¼ cup) soft light brown sugar
½ tsp ground cinnamon
½ tbsp lemon juice
1 tbsp cornflour (cornstarch)
1 tsp vanilla extract

For the toffee sauce

120g (4oz) coconut cream
80g (3oz) soft light brown sugar
½ tbsp cornflour (cornstarch)
Pinch of smoked sea salt (optional)

To decorate

6 clean oak twigs
6 bay leaves

8. To fry the doughnuts, use a floured spatula to transfer one doughnut at a time to your hot oil and fry for about 2 minutes on each side until golden brown in colour. Remove with tongs and place on kitchen towel to soak up any excess oil. Before the doughnuts cool, roll in the remaining caster sugar and set aside while you make the filling.

9. Put all the ingredients for the filling into a saucepan and cook over a low heat for about 25 minutes, or until you have chunks of apple suspended in a silky sauce. Stir from time to time to make sure the apples don't catch on the bottom of the pan. Remove from the heat and allow to cool while you make the sauce.

10. In another small pan, heat the coconut cream, sugar and cornflour over a medium heat, stirring constantly. When the mixture begins to develop a foamy texture, lower the heat and continue stirring for 5 minutes. Add a pinch of smoked salt, if using. Remove from the heat and allow to cool.

11. Cut small crosses into the top of each doughnut. Put the filling into a piping bag fitted with a small nozzle and fill each doughnut with roughly one-sixth of the filling. Place a clean wooden twig and a leaf into the top (make sure the twig and leaf are both from a non-toxic plant). Drizzle over the toffee sauce and enjoy! These doughnuts should ideally be eaten within a few days of making them.

Crab apple and pumpkin soup

This wonderfully warming soup is hugely comforting as the weather gets chillier. With crab apple, pumpkin, maple, ginger and mixed spice, it tastes like an autumnal walk in the woods!

You can use your pumpkins left over from Samhain or Halloween celebrations for this recipe, but remember they're not grown for eating purposes and might lack the flavour that eating pumpkins have.

SERVES 2

450g (1lb) pumpkin or squash
1 tbsp olive oil, plus extra for drizzling
1 white onion, finely chopped
2 garlic cloves
½ tsp ground ginger
½ tsp ground mixed spice
200g (7oz) peeled, cored and cubed crab apples
300ml (1¼ cups) vegetable stock
80ml (⅓ cup) double cream, plus extra for drizzling
1 tsp maple syrup
1 tsp apple cider vinegar
Salt and freshly ground black pepper

1. Prepare your pumpkin by cutting into chunks and cutting away the tough skin and seedy membrane. Pick the seeds out and give them a good wash to remove any leftover flesh. Place on some kitchen towel and allow to dry.
2. Heat the olive oil in a large saucepan and add the onion. Fry for about 3 minutes until soft and translucent. Add the garlic, ginger and mixed spice and fry for another 2 minutes.
3. Add the pumpkin or squash chunks and continue to cook for about 5 minutes. Add the cubed crab apples and cook for another 5 minutes.
4. Pour the vegetable stock into the pan, bring to the boil and continue to simmer for about 10 minutes, or until you can easily push a fork through the apple and pumpkin chunks.
5. Stir in the double cream, maple syrup, vinegar, salt and pepper and blend with a hand blender until smooth. At this point you can pass through a sieve if you'd like it to be extra-smooth. Return to the pan to reheat before serving.

Recipe continues over the page

For the topping (optional)
Small gourd
    or pumpkin
1 tbsp soy sauce

6. To make the optional topping, preheat the oven to 200°C/400°F/gas 6. Cut the small gourd or pumpkin in half lengthways and score the flesh to create a diamond pattern. Drizzle with oil and sprinkle with salt. Roast in the oven for about 30 minutes until soft.
7. While the pumpkin is roasting, toast your pumpkin seeds in a dry pan over a medium heat for about 4 minutes, flipping occasionally, until golden and crunchy. In the last minute, drizzle over the soy sauce.
8. Scoop the roasted pumpkin into chunks and top the soup. Sprinkle over the pumpkin seeds and drizzle over extra double cream.

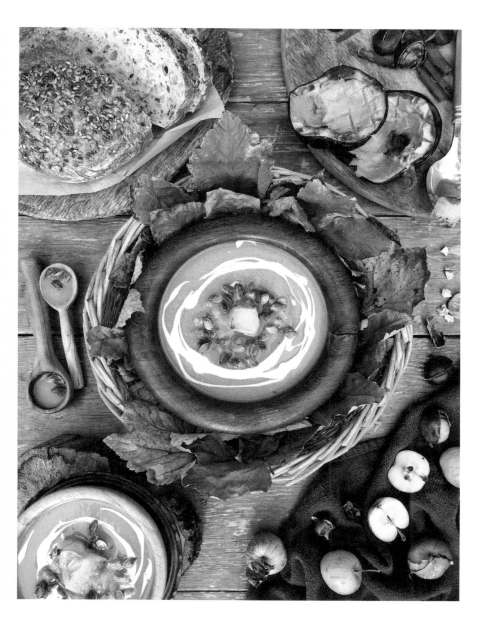

Blackberries

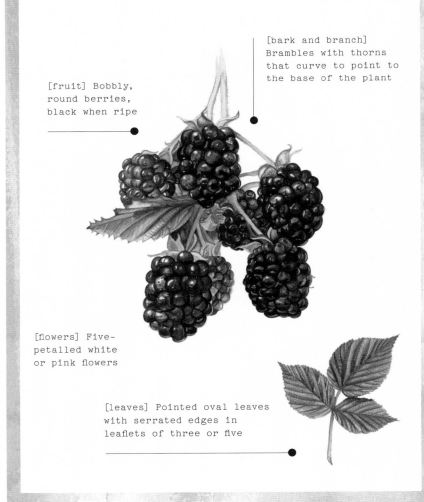

[bark and branch]
Brambles with thorns
that curve to point to
the base of the plant

[fruit] Bobbly,
round berries,
black when ripe

[flowers] Five-
petalled white
or pink flowers

[leaves] Pointed oval leaves
with serrated edges in
leaflets of three or five

Foraging notes

No good foraging book could be complete without mention of blackberries. They are the ultimate beginner-friendly wild fruit: a wholesome, juicy place where so many start their journeys. The memory, excitement and novelty of gobbling sweet berries from the hedgerows as children stay with many of us. I remember the alleyways we used to walk through on the way home from school became hives of activity when the blackberries ripened. We'd fill our hats, pockets and book bags with treasure. I can almost see our parents' dismay as we emptied our grubby pockets of squished berries and asked for crumble!

You'll find blackberries waiting for you in hedgerows and scrappy corners of land throughout September. Easily identified and with no toxic lookalikes that might confuse, look for thickets of thorny brambles, with little bobbly berries. The berries begin their lives bright green, mature into red (which might make some people think they've found wild raspberries) and then ripen into deep purple/black berries.

Once you've collected a lovely little basket of ripe blackberries, head home to make yourself a comforting jar of jam, a nostalgic crumble, or for something a little different, how about blackberry and balsamic glaze to drizzle over meat, grilled halloumi, or tofu (see page 233 and replace elderberries with blackberries)?

Blackberry recipes

Blackberries differ from each other hugely in flavour depending on subspecies and environment, so before cooking with blackberries, make sure you've tasted one to gauge its sweetness.

Blackberries are easy to pick but can hide a lot of little bugs. I'm not overly fussed about a bit of extra protein but will give them a good clean if I'm making food for others. I find the best way to get bugs out of blackberries is to fill a bowl with 4 parts cold water to 1 part vinegar and then add the blackberries. Swirl the blackberries around for a few moments until the bugs float to the surface. Scoop them up with a spoon or cup and release them into the garden. Let the blackberries air dry before you use them.

Plant lore, folk medicine & magic

Much of the English folklore surrounding blackberries can be translated into quite practical advice on when they're best eaten. It's said that after 29 September, the devil wees or spits on the blackberries so they should be left. In other places, it's said that after that date the blackberries belong to the witches, and taking them will stir up anger and put you at risk of being cursed. Whatever the tale, blackberries are certainly sweeter before October.

There are also some strange and quite wonderful blackberry traditions that were historically thought of as medicinal. Childhood diseases such as whooping cough and rheumatism were thought to be cured by passing children under boughs of blackberry brambles, sometimes repeating prayers and sometimes while the child ate half a slice of bread and butter. The other half would be given to a bird and when the bird ate the bread, the child would be cured.

Blackberry chocolate pots

Blackberry and chocolate is such a wonderful and undervalued combination. I love these little decadent pots, especially because they're made with whole foods and are much better for you than shop-bought ones. If you're cooking for a crowd, you could also use the filling to pour into a pastry case and make a blackberry chocolate tart!

MAKES 6–8

Approx. 100g (3½oz) blackberries, plus a few to decorate
2 tbsp plus 1 tsp maple syrup
3 tbsp water
100g (3½oz) dark chocolate, plus shavings to decorate
250ml (1 cup) full-fat coconut milk
1 tbsp coconut oil
½ tsp vanilla extract
25g (⅓ cup) cacao powder

1. Put the blackberries, 1 teaspoon maple syrup and water into a small frying pan. Heat over a low-medium heat for about 3 minutes, then squash half of the blackberries with the back of a fork. Set aside for later.

2. Grate or finely chop your dark chocolate and put into a large bowl.

3. Heat the coconut milk, coconut oil and 2 tablespoons maple syrup in a saucepan until very hot (close to, but not quite boiling.) Remove from the heat, add the vanilla extract and stir to combine.

4. Pour the coconut milk mixture over the chocolate, cover and leave for about 3 minutes, or until the chocolate has melted.

5. Give the chocolate and coconut mixture a good stir – it should be glossy and smooth. (If you have unmelted chocolate pieces left, microwave in 5-second bursts, stirring after each go, until there are no more chocolate chunks.)

6. Gently stir in the cacao powder until combined and then add the blackberry mixture; don't overmix, just swirl the blackberries through.

7. Divide the mixture between little pots or espresso cups and leave to set overnight.

8. Decorate with more blackberries and chocolate shavings.

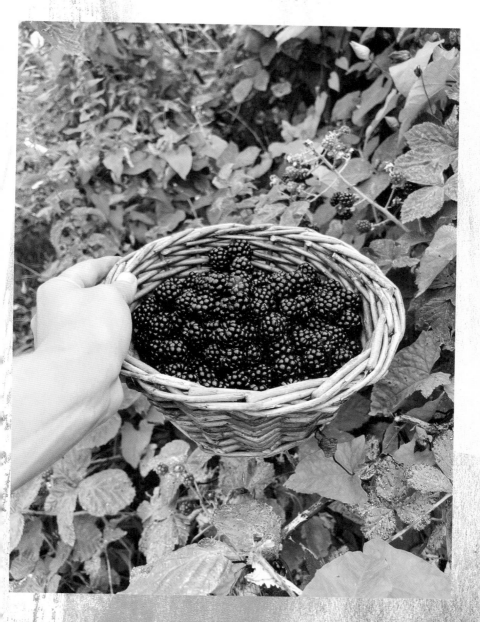

Blackberry crumble bars

This recipe is a delicious take on a classic crumble. Perfect for picnics and bring-a-dish parties, these have all the comfort and warmth of a crumble, without the mess! You can use all blackberries, or add in some elderberries, blackcurrants or blueberries for this recipe, depending on what you have and what's in season!

MAKES 9–12

For the base and topping
200g (1 cup) granulated sugar
1 tsp baking powder
375g (3 cups) plain (all-purpose) flour
¼ tsp salt
Finely grated zest of 1 small unwaxed lemon
225g (8oz) cold unsalted butter, cut into cubes
1 large egg, beaten
½ tsp vanilla extract

For the berry layer
600g (1lb 5oz) chopped fresh berries (or use frozen)
100g (½ cup) granulated sugar
4 tsp cornflour (cornstarch) (8tsp if using frozen berries)
Juice of 1 small lemon

1. Preheat the oven to 190°C/375°F/gas 5. Grease and line a 25cm (10in) square baking tin with parchment paper.
2. To make the base and topping, combine the sugar, baking powder, flour and salt in a large bowl. Add the lemon zest, butter, egg and vanilla and rub together with your fingertips until a fine crumble is formed.
3. Put all the berry layer ingredients into another bowl and mix! (If you are using frozen berries, double the quantity of cornflour.)
4. Put a little more than half of the crumble mixture into the base of the prepared pan and gently press down to form the base of your crumble bars.
5. Spread the filling over the crust and crumble the remaining dough over the top of the berries.
6. Bake for about 40 minutes, or until the top is light golden brown.
7. Transfer the tin to a wire rack to cool, before cutting into squares.

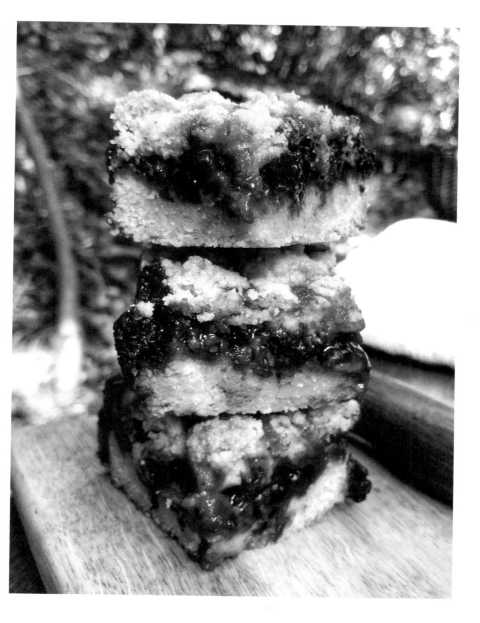

Hazelnut

[mature nut] Round,
hard brown shells with
a slightly flat top and
pointed fuzzy tip

[leaves] Pointed
circular leaves
with serrated
edges

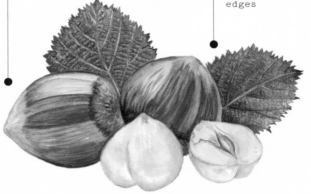

[immature nut] Soft
green nut, covered with
a green papery sheath

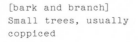

[bark and branch]
Small trees, usually
coppiced

Foraging notes

Hazelnuts are a wonderful autumnal treat and can be gathered straight from the tree, or picked up from the forest floor after a heavy wind has caused them to fall. They look just like the hazelnuts you can buy in shops, with round shells, half-covered by a papery sheath.

Brown, ripe nuts can be hard to find because the squirrels and mice love them so much! Hazelnuts can be eaten fresh and green but they're more flavoursome when they're brown; harvesting them when they're green and almost ripe, leaving them in an airing cupboard for a few days should do it. When they're done, shell and roast for 20 minutes to bring out all the flavour.

After roasting, rub off the outer skins and then sprinkle over salads or soups, blend them with some cocoa powder and maple syrup for a wild 'Nutella' (see page 195) or stir them into pancakes or granola for a delightfully wild breakfast.

Hazelnut recipes

It's so easy to make something delicious and rich with hazelnuts. They simply need harvesting, drying out and cracking open – a regular nut cracker works well. Once they're shelled I would always recommend roasting them to bring out their delicious flavour. Simply place in an oven preheated to 180°C/350°F/gas 4 for about 20 minutes. The skins will turn very dark and can be rubbed off when the nuts are cool. The nuts will be golden brown and delicious.

Plant lore, folk medicine & magic

In Celtic mythology, the hazel was an incredibly important and holy tree. It symbolised wisdom, poetry and knowledge and features heavily in folklore. One particular tale is the tale of the nine holy hazels, of which there are many versions. My favourite is an Irish version, which is also the origin story of Fionn mac Cumhaill, a mythical hunter-warrior in Irish mythology.

In this story there was a magical well, sometimes known as the well of life. The nuts from the nine holy hazels that overhung the well would drop into the water. Salmon would eat the nuts and any person who consumed one of these salmon would become all-knowing.

A master druid caught one of these salmon and demanded that his apprentice cook it for him. He also warned that the cook would be severely punished if he ate any of it. The boy heated a pan over the fire and, dropping the salmon into the hot oil, the pan spat oil out at him and coated his thumb. To stop the burning, he put his thumb to his mouth and accidentally absorbed the magic of the hazel.

It wasn't only in Celtic mythology that hazels were documented as holy. A manuscript found in China from the year 2838 BC names the hazelnut as one of the five sacred nourishments God bestowed on human beings. The hazel is also known to be a symbol of love and fertility. The Somerset saying 'plenty of catkins, plenty of prams' refers to the folkloric idea that when the hazel catkins are plentiful, there will be lots of babies born.

Wild 'Nutella'

This creamy, nutty and chocolatey spread is absolutely delicious slathered on toast and crumpets and even combined with hot milk to make a delicious warming drink.

MAKES 600ML

400g (14oz) roasted hazelnuts
1 tsp vanilla extract
½ tsp sea salt
100g (3½oz) dark chocolate, grated or finely chopped
1–2 tbsp maple syrup (optional)

1. Put the hazelnuts into a high-speed blender and blend on low-medium speed until you have a creamy and smooth nut butter – this should take about 8 minutes. Scrape down the sides as you go.
2. Add the vanilla and salt and blend again until combined.
3. Set a heatproof bowl over a saucepan of just simmering water, making sure the base of the bowl doesn't touch the water. Add the chocolate and stir until melted.
4. Scrape the melted chocolate into the blender and blend again until combined. Taste your 'Nutella', and add maple syrup to taste, if using.
5. Transfer to a sterilised jar. Stored at room temperature, this spread will last for up to 3 weeks.

Wild 'Nutella' loaf cake

This cake has been a go-to pudding for my autumn workshops for the last few years. It's incredibly easy to make and lashings of wild 'Nutella' on top make it beyond delicious. Orange juice helps the cake to rise and makes it a little more autumnal.

MAKES 1 LARGE LOAF CAKE

250ml (1 cup) oat milk
Juice of 1 large orange
320g (2½ cups) plain (all-purpose) flour
200g (1 cup) caster (superfine) sugar
1 tsp baking powder
Pinch of salt
100ml (3½fl oz) vegetable oil
150g (5oz) wild 'Nutella' (see page 195)

For the topping
200g (7oz) wild 'Nutella'
100g (¾ cup) roasted hazelnuts, chopped

1. Preheat the oven to 170°C/340°F/gas 3 and grease and line a 25cm (10in) loaf tin with parchment paper.
2. Combine the oat milk and orange juice in a jug (don't worry if it curdles). Sift the flour into a bowl, add the sugar, baking powder and salt and mix well.
3. Add the oil to the milk mixture and stir, then pour the wet ingredients into the dry ingredients.
4. Fold in until just combined (don't overmix) then pour around a quarter of the cake batter into another bowl and combine with the wild 'Nutella'.
5. Pour the white batter into the prepared loaf tin and then distribute the brown batter over the top. Use a table knife to swirl the brown batter throughout.
6. Bake for 50 minutes–1 hour until golden and a skewer inserted comes out clean.
7. Remove from the oven and leave to cool in the tin for 5–10 minutes before removing from the tin and transferring to a wire rack to cool completely.
8. Once the cake is cool, spread over the wild 'Nutella' for the topping and sprinkle over the chopped roasted hazelnuts.

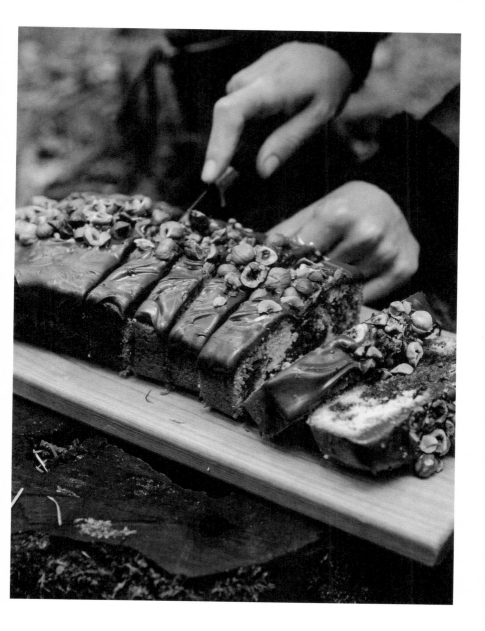

Acorn

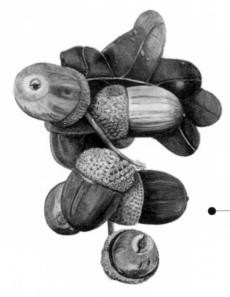

[bark and branch] Light grey-brown bark with deep fissures and ridges

[nuts] Smooth, oval nut with a pointed tip, sitting in a cup called a a 'cupule'

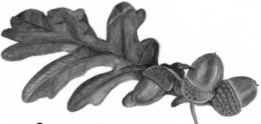

[leaves] Distinctive leaves with long 'lobes' and deep 'sinuses'

Foraging notes

Grand old oaks produce such a bounty of beautiful acorns, but aside from the caps being used for fairy hats, they're rarely taken home and put to good use. It often surprises people that you can eat acorns, but historically they've been an important food source. They're incredible high in protein, healthy fat, B vitamins, magnesium and fibre and would have kept many ancient civilisations healthy and well fed.

Acorns are high in tannins, which makes them inedible in their raw form, but after going through a process called leaching, they are delicious, nutty and unique (some say similar to chestnuts, but of course they have their own flavour). To leach an acorn, it must be shelled, crushed and allowed to soak in water to draw out the tannins.

Ancient people had ingenious ways of doing this; they would dig huge pits near fresh running rivers and fill them with acorns. The water in the earth would draw out the tannins and the people would return a year later, to harvest their acorns and bury a fresh batch. The acorns would be washed and eaten fresh or allowed to dry for later consumption. Don't worry, I won't be asking you to find your nearest river for these upcoming recipes!

Acorn recipes

Once processed, acorns can either be eaten as fresh nuts, roasted and sprinkled on salads, ground down and used as a coffee substitute or as a flour to make cakes, breads and biscuits.

When you're harvesting your acorns make sure they are brown and evenly coloured all over. Also check they don't have any little holes in the nut, as these are weevil holes and you'll be sure to find one in the acorn!

Plant lore, folk medicine & magic

The acorn, like the mighty oak it grows from, is a symbol of strength and power, as well as perseverance and hard work. This symbolism around power and strength has been a theme throughout military history and can still be seen today. Roman generals were gifted crowns of oak leaves on return from victorious battles and today in the US armed forces a small bronze twig, bearing four oak leaves and three acorns, is worn on the ribbon of medals to signify the wearer has a second award of that same medal.

The acorn and the oak also have strong ties to lightning and the divine. Because of their size oaks are most likely to be struck by lightning, yet can often to continue to grow after a strike. Ancient druids believed that it was through this lightning that the gods delivered mistletoe, which was a powerful medicine and which would be harvested by a priest.

In Norse folklore, it's said that the god of war, Thor, once took refuge from a devastating storm under an oak tree. To this day, in some parts of Norway and Scandinavia it's believed that putting an acorn on your windowsill or wearing one as a pendant will help protect home and family from being struck by lightning.

Acorn flour

This recipe takes you through the entire process of leaching your acorns and turning them into a flour to be used like a spelt flour. If you're making breads and cakes, you'll want to use it alongside a white flour. Although 100% acorn flour bread is historically interesting, it's not well suited to our modern-day palates, but even by using smaller percentages, you can create a nutrient-packed bake.

MAKES APPROX. 400G (14OZ)

1.5kg (3lb 5oz) acorns

1. Preheat the oven to 170°C/340°F/gas 3.
2. Put the acorns into a bowl of water, discarding any that float (this will get rid of any that may have weevils).
3. Drain the acorns, dry them with a clean tea towel and spread them on a baking tray. Bake in the oven for 10 minutes (this helps the skin separate from the nut before processing).
4. Bash each acorn with a hammer to split the shell (this is much easier to do if you hold the acorn upright, so it's taller). Then remove the shell and peel off any brown skin.
5. Now it's time to leach the acorns of their tannins. This can be done with hot or cold water, but cold water keeps more of the oils and starches in.
6. Put the acorns in a blender and top up with water until the maximum fill point on your blender is reached. Blend on high speed for a few minutes and then strain through a muslin cloth.
7. Keeping your acorn meal in the muslin cloth, tie it up and run under a cold tap until the water runs clear. Squish and move the acorn meal around in the cloth under the running water for 6–10 minutes, or until the water runs clear.

Recipe continues over the page

(Alternatively, you can put the acorn meal in a clean jar, top up with water and cover with a muslin cloth. Twice a day for four days, strain off the water and top up with fresh water. When it's done, the acorn meal will not taste bitter.)

8. When you're done leaching, drain the acorn meal and use the muslin cloth to squeeze as much water out as possible

9. Preheat the oven to 150°C/300°F/gas 2. Tip the acorn meal on to a baking tray and put into the oven for about 30 minutes, or until it is nice and dark in colour and tastes nutty. At this stage you can use the meal like any other roasted nut, for making my acorn truffles on page 204 or for making acorn coffee.

10. The meal can now be ground into a flour with a pestle and mortar or using a high-speed blender.

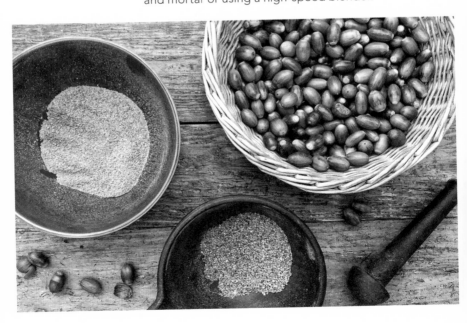

Acorn pancakes

You can use your acorn flour for breads, cakes and biscuits, but these simple pancakes are my favourite. After all the work you've put into making your acorn flour, these pancakes will be a real treat!

MAKES 8

75g (2½oz) acorn
flour (see
page 201)
75g (2½oz) self-
raising flour
1 tsp baking powder
1 tbsp sugar
Pinch of salt
1 tbsp vanilla extract
400ml (14fl oz) plant-
based milk
Oil, for frying

1. Combine the acorn flour and self-raising flour in a bowl, then add baking powder, sugar and the pinch of salt and stir to combine. Add the vanilla extract and then slowly pour in the milk until you get a smooth, thick batter.
2. In a frying pan, heat 1 teaspoon oil and swirl to coat the bottom of the pan. Pour little circles of batter on to the surface of the pan (you should be able to fit in 2–3 in one go).
3. When you can see little bubbles appearing on the top side of the pancakes, flip them over and cook for another 2–3 minutes, or until cooked through.
4. Create a pancake stack and top with your favourite fruits and toppings. How about blackberries and some immunity-boosting elderberry syrup (see page 231)?

Acorn truffles

These little truffles are so worth the time spent making them. They're melt-in-the-mouth and super-chocolatey with a delicious crunch from the acorn meal and a touch of salt from the pretzel stick stems! Perfect for a post-mushroom hunt woodland treat! Make sure you serve these at room temperature.

MAKES 6

150g (5oz) dark chocolate
3 tbsp coconut milk
2 tbsp acorn meal (not ground) (see page 201)
2 pretzel sticks

1. Grate or finely chop 100g (3½oz) of the dark chocolate and put into a large bowl.
2. Heat the coconut milk in a saucepan until very hot but not quite boiling.
3. Pour the coconut milk over the chocolate, cover and leave for around 3 minutes, or until the chocolate has melted.
4. Give the chocolate and coconut mixture a good stir; it should be glossy and smooth. If you have unmelted chocolate pieces left, microwave for in 5-second bursts, stirring after each go, until there are no more chocolate chunks.
5. Put the mixture in the fridge for 2–3 hours. This setting time is really important for shaping your truffles. If you leave it too long, it will be too firm to shape. A good test is to insert a knife, it should come out mostly clean.
6. Using a teaspoon, scoop out one portion of chocolate at a time and mould with wet hands into acorn shapes.
7. Melt the remaining 50g (2oz) dark chocolate in a small heatproof bowl set over a pan of just simmering water (or in the microwave) and dip the acorn tops into the chocolate. Finally, sprinkle acorn meal over the chocolate.
8. Snap the pretzel sticks into short acorn 'stems' and push them into the top of the acorn truffles. Leave the acorn truffles to set.

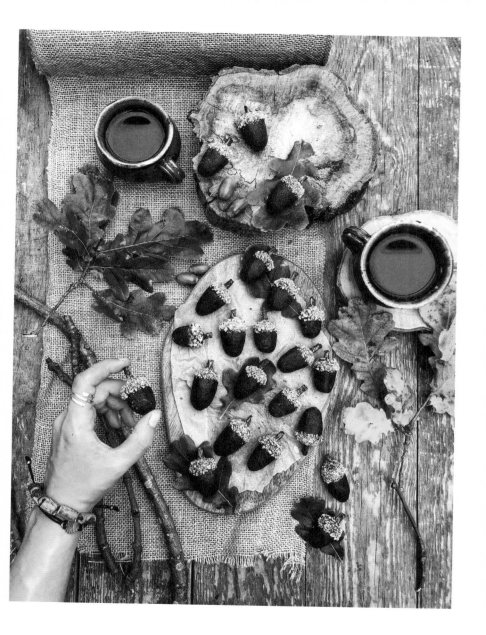

Hawthorn

[bark and branch] Trees with grey, knotted bark

[leaves] Five pointed leaves

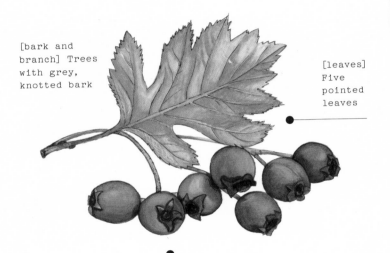

[fruit] Small, round red fruit with a stone inside; five-pointed star on the bottom of the berry

[flowers] White to pink blossom, with a very odd 'meaty' smell!

Foraging notes

Hawthorn is one of most common, most undervalued hedgerow plants we have access to. Most English hedgerows will have at least a few hawthorns. They were once planted up in huge numbers as common land became private land and hedgerows began to divide the country. They were selected (along with blackthorn) for their thick and thorny protective properties, to keep animals in and strangers out.

The berries, picked straight from the tree, taste almost like a savoury apple and have a creamy texture, similar to a ripe avocado – not the most pleasant snack, but when you know what to do with them, they can be a wonderful ingredient!

The hawthorn produces the strangest-smelling blossom in spring, which smells vaguely like rotting meat. The young spring leaves were once such a staple for poor folk that they came to be known as 'bread and cheese'. They do make quite a lovely addition to a salad! The best bit by far is, of course, the berry.

Hawthorn recipes

To make something delicious with your hawthorn berries, it's important you pick them when they're ripe. They're ready to harvest when they're dark red and when the flesh comes away from the stone easily when squashed between finger and thumb.

Plant lore, folk medicine & magic

Hawthorn trees are often seen as stand-alone, windswept trees, especially in Cornwall and Ireland. This echoes their magical importance throughout history on the British Isles. The hawthorn tree was believed to be the home of fairies and the gateway between this realm and the realm of divine higher beings. The fairies guarding this gateway would smite and seek revenge on anyone who cut down or harmed the tree in any way ... so any labourer asked to clear a field of trees would have left the hawthorns well alone!

Fairies were not the sweet and angelic creatures depicted in many modern-day tales. They were originally mischievous at best and evil at worse. Stories of fairies stealing babies and making people dance around fairy rings until their feet bled made them fairly ferocious beings not to be messed with. Warnings never to fall asleep under a hawthorn tree, lest you be carried away by the fairies were plentiful.

In traditional and modern herbalism, hawthorn is known to be good for the heart and for circulation on a physical and energetic level.

Hawthorn and honey fruit roll ups

Fruit roll ups bring me so much joy. They remind me of a snack we used to have in our lunchboxes called Winders. These ones might not come with the comic on the paper (although you could always draw your own) but they're just as delicious and free from sugar and plastic packaging!

You can make fruit roll ups with any fruit so long as you can make it into a purée. This recipe works wonderfully with plums and blackberries too.

MAKES 12

800g (1¾lb) hawthorns, stripped from the branch and with any bits of stem removed
500g (1lb 2oz) apples, peeled, cored and cubed
3 tbsp lemon juice
Few sprigs of thyme or a handful of honeysuckle flowers (optional)
170g (6oz) honey

1. Line two baking sheets with parchment paper and preheat the oven to its lowest setting, 110°C/230°F/ gas ¼. (Alternatively, if you have a dehydrator use two silicone dehydrating trays and set the dehydrator to a medium setting.)
2. Put the hawthorns, apples, lemon juice, thyme leaves or honeysuckle flowers, if using, into a large, heavy-based saucepan and cook over a low heat for about 30 minutes until you are left with a thick fruit pulp.
3. Put a sieve over a large bowl and pass the mixture through the sieve in two batches (to avoid overloading the sieve). Press the mixture through with the back of a spoon to get as much fruit purée as possible.
4. Add the honey and stir to combine.
5. Pour half of the fruit purée on to one of your lined baking sheets (or silicone trays), then spread the mixture out evenly with a spatula or spoon until it is a few millimetres thick. Repeat with the other half of the fruit purée on the second tray.
6. Put into the oven (or dehydrator) and leave for 12–15 hours, or until the fruit purée is dried out and has reached a leathery consistency.
7. Cut the paper and dried fruit purée into long, thin strips. Roll these strips and secure with a little food-safe string. Your fruit roll ups can be stored in an airtight jar for up to 6 months.

Hawthorn ketchup

Hawthorn ketchup is one of my favourite things to make in autumn. I love knowing that I'm putting those little berries to good use and making them the star of the show for a change. You can use it as a dipping sauce, as the base of a pizza or pasta sauce, or as an ingredient for more complex sauces such as sweet and sour or BBQ sauce.

You could also add various spices, chilli and other fruits to this recipe. How about a handful of blackberries or some warming mixed spice?

MAKES APPROX. 2 JARS

600g (1lb 5oz) hawthorns, stripped from the branch and with any bits of stem removed
400ml (14fl oz) water
300ml (1¼ cups) apple cider vinegar
190g (1 cup) granulated sugar

1. Give your hawthorns a rinse and then add them to a large saucepan with the water and apple cider vinegar. Bring to the boil, then turn the heat down and simmer for around 30 minutes, or until you're left with a thick, fruity pulp. You may need to add more water as you continue to simmer the mixture.
2. When it's ready, you should be able to see that the hawthorn flesh coming away from the stones and it should be thick enough that a spoon leaves a trail when you stir the mixture.
3. Put a sieve over a large bowl and pass the mix through the sieve in two batches (to avoid overloading the sieve). Press the mixture down through the sieve with the back of a spoon to get as much fruit purée as possible.
4. In the bowl, you should have what looks like tomato purée. Put this back into a clean saucepan and add the sugar. (Remember that hawthorns will all differ in taste and sweetness. You may need to add more or less sugar, until the sauce reaches your preferred sweetness.)
5. Transfer to sterilised jars while still warm and seal tightly. This will last for up to a year before the jar is opened. Once opened, it will last up to a month in the fridge. It also freezes very well.

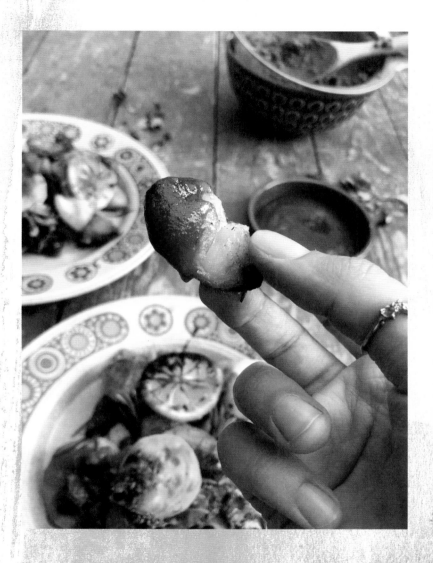

Parasol Mushroom

[stipe] Creamy white stipe with a brown snakeskin
effect. Ring around the stipe is large, soft and
cottony. It can be broken off easily and moved up
and down the stipe. Bulbous at the base

[porous
underside] White
to cream gills

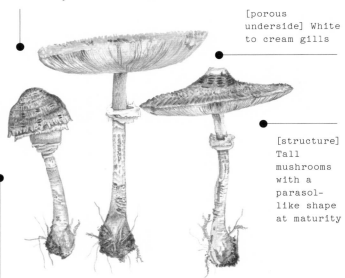

[structure]
Tall
mushrooms
with a
parasol-
like shape
at maturity

[cap] Tan in colour with brown
scales growing in concentric circles
around the cap. Up to 30cm (12in)
across. When young, the caps are
round, flattening out with maturity
and eventually pointing like tipis

Foraging notes

Parasol mushrooms are hard to miss as they're incredibly tall and are usually found growing in grassland where they're easily visible. They start their lives looking faintly similar to lollipops, with a tall stem holding a closed mushroom cap in the shape of a little ball. Then as the cap opens out, they begin to look like little tipis and eventually open out to resemble dinner plates. They grow in abundance, and you'll usually find 30–40 growing in one patch. You'll only need a few to make something delicious and, as always, you should leave any with a closed cap to open out and spread their spores.

The caps have a cottony, soft feel to them and also smell like warm milk. They're beautiful simply fried with butter but will reduce substantially in size when cooked.

Parasol mushroom recipes

Before using your parasol mushroom, remove the tough stipe (stem) from the cap and use it for something else. I like to throw them in a soup or stock. Stems can also be dried if you have a dehydrator and then blended to make a flavoursome mushroom stock powder. The texture of the cap is nice and meaty and the flavour mild and mushroomy!

Mushroom safety

Parasols are so great for beginners because as long as you make sure you pick them when they're big (with caps at least 12cm/5in across), there's really nothing you could get them confused with!

The reason we pick them big is to avoid mistaking them for the very dangerous Lepiota genus – also known as the dapperlings. Even if you're sure you're in a parasol patch – leave those little ones alone! To be 100 per cent sure you have a parasol, make sure your mushroom is growing in meadow or field, has a snakeskin stipe, a fleecy cream cap with brown patches, a point on the top and a big fluffy ring around the stipe that can be moved up and down!

If you have something that looks very similar but much shaggier, or fleecier, you've got a shaggy parasol! These are also edible but don't agree with everyone, so (as always with wild mushrooms) cook one and just have a little first to see how you go!

Parasol mushroom ravioli

This is hands-down my favourite mushroom recipe. I've made it with all kinds of mushrooms, from parasols, to field mushrooms to chanterelles. There's really not many mushrooms it doesn't work with! In my humble opinion, there's nothing like freshly made pasta, but when it's stuffed with wild mushrooms, delicious weeds and drowning in truffle sauce it's on a whole other level. Heavenly.

**MAKES 2 LARGE OR
4 SMALL PORTIONS**

For the pasta dough
300g (2¼ cups)
  00 flour, plus extra
  for dusting
4 medium eggs
1 tbsp olive oil

For the filling
1 tbsp olive oil
1 onion, finely diced
300g (10oz)
  mushrooms,
  finely diced
1 garlic clove, grated
  or finely chopped
10 nettle tops
  (or use spinach)
Small handful of
  ground ivy leaves
  (see page 72)
250g (9oz) ricotta
  (or use vegan
  soft cheese)
Salt and freshly
  ground black
  pepper

1. To make the pasta dough, make a mountain of flour on a clean work surface and then make a well in the centre. Crack your eggs into the well and add the olive oil. Whisk up the eggs and oil and then begin to incorporate the flour until the whole thing is combined.
2. If making pasta by hand, knead the dough for around 10 minutes, then place in the fridge to chill for 20 minutes while you make the filling. If you're using a pasta maker, skip the kneading and just leave the dough to chill in the fridge.
3. Heat the olive oil in a frying pan; when hot, add the onion and soften for around 4 minutes.
4. Add the diced mushrooms and fry for a further 3 minutes before adding the garlic and frying for a further minute. Remove from the heat. Steam your nettle tops for about 3 minutes, or until dark green and slightly wilted. Then plunge into a bowl of ice-cold water to stop them cooking more. Remove and drain, then pick the nettle leaves off the stems and chop them finely together with the ground ivy.
5. Add the chopped nettle, ground ivy, ricotta and a generous pinch of salt and pepper to your mushrooms and stir well to combine. Set aside while you make your pasta.
6. Remove the pasta dough from the fridge and divide into four pieces. Pat the dough into roughly a square shape and generously dust your work surface and pasta machine with flour.

Recipe continues over the page

For the pasta sauce

1 tbsp olive oil
1 white onion,
    finely chopped
1 garlic clove,
    crushed
250ml (1 cup) double
    (heavy) cream
½ tsp freshly
    grated nutmeg
Handful of grated
    Parmesan cheese,
    plus extra to serve
1 fresh truffle, plus
    extra to serve
Salt and freshly
    ground black
    pepper

Set your pasta machine to its widest setting and run the dough through six or seven times, folding after each time. This is the kneading process. (If you are making pasta by hand, skip this step and roll out your pasta with a rolling pin until only a few millimetres thick. Then cut in half down the middle so you have two strips of pasta. Continue from step 8)

7. Now progressively set your pasta machine to a thinner setting, while keeping it well floured. Do not fold the pasta any more. When you reach the thinnest setting, you will have one long strip of very thin pasta. Cut it in half down the middle so you have two shorter lengths of pasta.

8. Place a teaspoon of filling at intervals along one of your pasta strips, so when you put your cutter over the filling, you can see a clear ring of pasta around the outside (this will form the edge of your pasta).

9. Now drape the other pasta strip over the first and press down around the filling. Press down gently to minimise any air between the two sheets of pasta and make sure the ravioli are sealed.

10. Now use a cookie cutter to cut out your pasta shapes.

11. Bring a large saucepan of water to the boil and cook the ravioli for 2–3 minutes, or until the pasta is cooked.

12. Meanwhile, make the sauce: heat the oil in a frying pan and fry the onion and garlic for a minute or until fragrant, then add the cream, nutmeg and salt and pepper.

13. Bring to a simmer, then turn off the heat and add the Parmesan. When the cheese has melted, grate in about 1 teaspoon of fresh truffle and stir to combine.

14. Drain the ravioli and toss gently in the sauce. Serve with extra Parmesan and grated truffle.

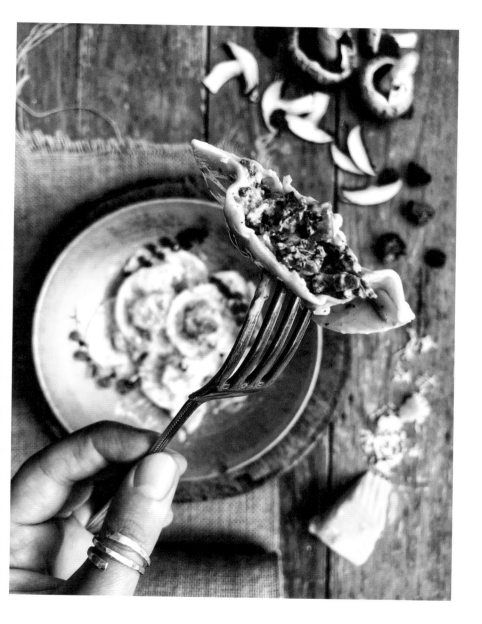

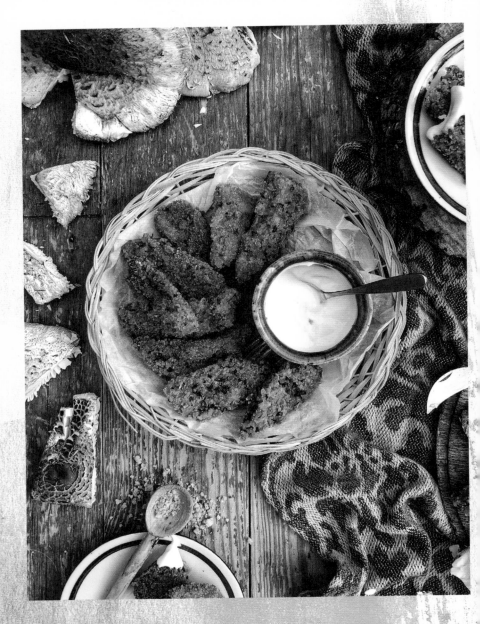

Parasol mushroom goujons

These herby, crunchy mushroom goujons are so good. As in, good enough to put your chicken nuggets in the bin. We make these deliciously crispy, herby breadcrumbed morsels hiding perfectly cooked, meaty mushroom whenever we find parasols and when they're out of season, we use portobello mushrooms. Serve with a lemon garlic mayonnaise for extra goodness.

These goujons can be made ahead of time and frozen before they are fried. Fry from frozen.

MAKES APPROX. 30

½ small loaf of sourdough bread (or any stale bread in the cupboard)
1 tsp finely ground sea salt
1 tbsp finely chopped herbs, such as ground ivy (see page 72) or rosemary
2 eggs (for a vegan substitute, use 90g/½ cup of chickpea flour mixed with 125ml/½ cup plant milk)
60g (½ cup) plain (all-purpose) flour
2 large parasol caps
Vegetable oil, for frying

1. Preheat the oven to 180°C/350°F/gas 4.
2. Break the bread into small chunks and arrange them on a baking tray in a single layer. Bake for around 15 minutes, or until golden brown and crispy. Remove from the oven and allow to cool completely, then blitz in a food processor until you have breadcrumbs.
3. Add the salt and herbs to the breadcrumbs and stir to combine. Put this in a bowl and put aside.
4. In another bowl, break the eggs and whisk with a fork. (For the vegan alternative, simply combine the flour and plant milk.) Place the flour in another bowl.
5. Cut the mushroom caps into rough goujon shapes, around 6–7cm (2–3in) in length.
6. Put a few centimetres of oil into a high-sided frying pan and heat over a medium-high heat until a crumb sizzles when dropped in.
7. Create an assembly line and move your mushrooms down the line, coating the mushrooms chunks first in flour, then in egg and finally in breadcrumbs. When the mushrooms are coated, add them to the oil, working in batches so you don't overcrowd the pan.
8. Cook each goujon for around 2–3 minutes on all four sides until golden brown and crispy all over. Remove with a slotted spoon and drain on kitchen paper.

Penny Bun Mushroom

[cap] Chestnut brown and up
to 25cm (10in) across

[structure]
Bulbous mushrooms
with a fat stipe
and convex cap

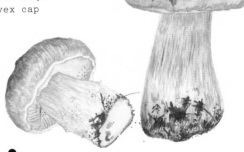

[porous underside]
Tight sponge texture
instead of gills,
creamy white to yellow
in colour

[stipe] Bulbous,
usually thicker
at the base, and
creamy white

Foraging notes

A penny bun, by any other name, would taste just as good! And there's lots of names to choose from, including cep, porcini, *Boletes edulus* and king bolete. Whatever you want to call them, they are one of the most highly prized edibles available to the forager, usually found growing from the earth around oak or pine trees.

One of the reasons why these are so valued is because they are firm and meaty with the most wonderful flavour. They also grow to a huge size, meaning you can get a pretty decent meal from just one of them. If you find loads, you can dry them and rehydrate them later to make a powerfully flavoured mushroom stock, or blitz the dried mushroom to a powder and use the powder for an umami hit or just to make any dish more powerfully mushroomy. The possibilities are endless.

Penny bun recipes

Penny buns are one of the most fantastic-tasting and versatile mushrooms on offer to the forager. Even when simply fried in butter, allowed to slightly caramelised in the pan and sprinkled with salt, it's an absolute pleasure to eat. Here are a few more of my favourite recipes for when we come across a good haul of penny buns.

Mushroom safety

Ceps are very beginner-friendly because they are in the bolete family, whose members are mostly edible with just a few poisonous ones. It's a great family to learn about because all the members (about 80 species in the UK) are easy to recognise and, with just two rules, you can eliminate the few poisonous species. The edible species are generally large, meaty and delicious!

For foraging purposes, we can consider any mushroom growing from the earth (and not the side of a tree) with a stipe and a porous underside a member of the bolete family – easy-peasy!

If you are sure you have a member of the bolete family (a mushroom with a bulbous stipe and porous underside) you can now use these two rules to make sure you have an edible one:

- If you can see any red on the mushroom, eliminate it!
- If you cut the mushroom and it stains blue, eliminate it!

Any bolete you are left with, is edible – hooray!

You might miss out on a few edible members of the bolete family by following these rules, but you'll also rule out all the toxic ones, so it's a great go-to rule if you don't want to learn every single member of the family and you want to find some yummy edible boletes! How handy is that?!

In terms of potential lookalikes, they are all members of the bolete family and are all safe to eat providing you follow the two rules above.

Red wine mushrooms with polenta

If you're looking for something comforting to make with your foraged mushrooms, look no further! Creamy, buttery polenta with rich, meaty mushrooms, swimming in a red wine gravy. If you fancy changing up this recipe a little, you could try polenta chips, mashed potato or even jacket potato, which is especially good if you're cooking over a campfire!

MAKES ENOUGH FOR 2 HUNGRY PEOPLE

For the mushrooms
4 tbsp butter
1 red onion, thinly sliced
500g (1lb 2oz) penny bun mushroom (or any other meaty mushroom of your choice – chanterelle, field mushroom, chestnut, shitake would all work well), sliced
5–7 sprigs of thyme
4 garlic cloves, crushed
1 tsp cornflour (cornstarch)
100ml (3½floz) good red wine
400ml (14fl oz) vegetable, chicken or mushroom stock

1. Make the polenta first by bringing the water to the boil with the salt in a large saucepan. When the water is boiling, pour the polenta slowly into the water, whisking constantly.
2. When all the polenta has been combined reduce the heat to a gentle simmer and continue to whisk until the polenta begins to thicken: this should take about 5 minutes and there should be no lumps in the polenta.
3. Cover the pan with a lid and cook for 25–30 minutes, stirring every 5 minutes. When the polenta is creamy and no longer grainy, remove from the heat.
4. Meanwhile, cook your mushrooms. Melt 2 tablespoons of the butter in a large, heavy-based frying pan, add the onion and soften for about 4 minutes.
5. Add the sliced mushrooms and thyme and fry for about 5 minutes over a high heat until the mushrooms are browned and slightly caramelised on the edges, then add the crushed garlic and fry for another minute.
6. Push the mushrooms aside and add the remaining butter. Stir the cornflour into the butter to make a paste and cook for a minute.
7. Add the wine and combine with the butter and cornflour. Cook for another minute before adding the stock and mushroom ketchup. Stir the whole thing to combine.

Recipe continues over the page

1 tbsp mushroom
    ketchup (or
    Worcestershire
    sauce)
Salt and freshly
    ground black
    pepper

For the polenta
1 litre (4 cups) water
1 tsp fine sea salt
160g (1 cup) polenta
3 tbsp butter
50g (½ cup) grated
    Parmesan cheese
    (or use a plant-
    based alternative)

8. Stir until the gravy has thickened and add salt and pepper to taste. When the gravy is thick and glossy, take off the heat.
9. Add the butter and cheese to the polenta and whip into the polenta for a good few minutes. Add salt and pepper to taste.
10. To serve, divide the polenta between two bowls and top with the mushrooms and gravy.

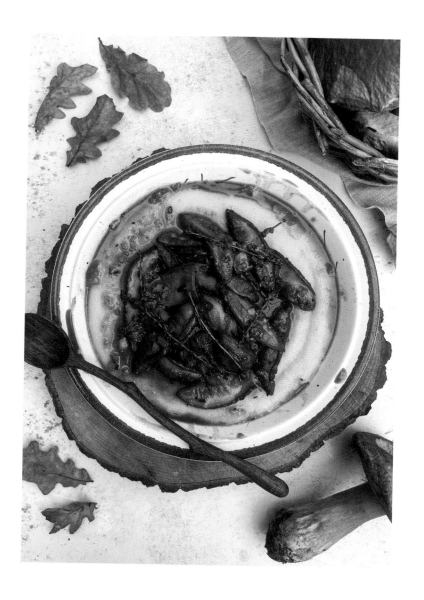

Mushrooms rolls

A meaty, mushroomy filling, packed with flavour and wrapped in buttery, flaky pastry. What could be better for an autumnal picnic? Serve with hawthorn ketchup (see page 210) for an extra dose of wild flavour.

MAKES 12

3 tbsp olive oil
2 white onions, chopped
6 garlic cloves, finely chopped
2 tbsp butter
900g (2lb) diced penny buns (or other meaty wild mushroom)
10 sprigs of thyme, leaves picked
8 tbsp soy sauce
4 tbsp mushroom ketchup (or Worcestershire sauce)
Large handful of curly parsley, chopped
130g (1 cup) roasted hazelnuts
2–3 tbsp vegan cheese (or nutritional yeast)
1 sheet of ready-rolled puff pastry
3 tbsp oat milk

1. Preheat the oven to 200°C/400°F/gas 6.
2. Heat 1 tablespoon of the oil in a frying pan and add the chopped onions. Cook over a low-medium heat until the onions are soft and golden brown, about 5 minutes. Stir in the chopped garlic and cook for a further minute. Remove from the heat and set aside.
3. Heat the remaining oil and the butter in a separate large frying pan. When the butter is melted add the mushrooms and thyme. Cook over a medium-high heat for about 10 minutes, allowing the mushrooms to caramelise and brown at the edges. Add a pinch of salt in the last minute.
4. Add the soy sauce and mushroom ketchup and cook for another few minutes until the mushrooms have absorbed the liquid. Stir through the parsley and cook for another minute, then take off the heat.
5. Blitz the hazelnuts in a food processor until they reach the texture of coarse breadcrumbs, then stir into the mushroom mixture along with the onion and garlic mixture and the vegan cheese; set aside.
6. To assemble the mushroom rolls, roll out the pastry and cut in half lengthways so you have two long strips of pastry.
7. Spoon half the mushroom mixture down the middle of each strip of pastry and brush one side of the pastry rectangle with oat milk.
8. Lift one long side of the pastry up and over the filling, then tuck and roll to create a tight roll. Cut them into shorter rolls – I like to cut each pastry strip into 4–6 pieces.

Salt and freshly
  ground black
  pepper
Sesame seeds,
  to garnish

9. Arrange the rolls on a baking tray, making sure they are seam side down. Cut a small diagonal slit in the top of each mushroom roll, then brush with the remaining oat milk and sprinkle with sesame seeds.

10. Bake in the oven for 20–25 minutes until the pastry is puffed up and golden brown. Serve hot from the oven, with hawthorn ketchup (see page 210). These are great cold too and will last up to 3 days in the fridge.

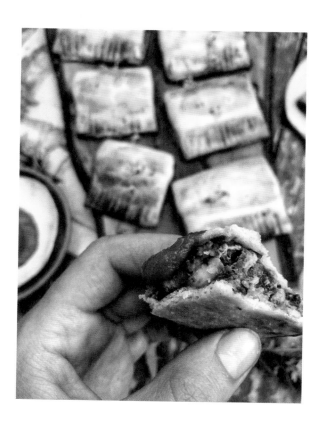

Elderberries

[leaves] Pointed oval
leaves in a leaf pattern
of two opposite pairs
and one pinnacle leaf

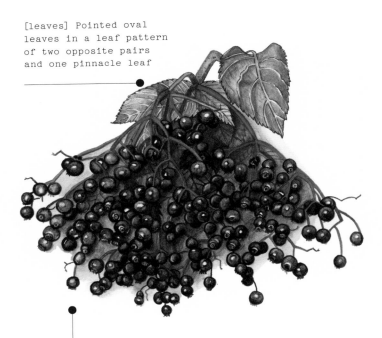

[fruit] Very small,
black berries which grow
in drooping clusters

[flowers] See
page 124

Foraging notes

We've already spoken about the magic of the elder and its flowers on page 125, but in the autumn, the Elder Mother will give us another gift, her elderberries – small, black berries bursting with dark juice and rich in vitamins. It's important to remember that the berries in their raw form are toxic, so should always be cooked before consumption. The stems, branches and leaves of the elder are mildly toxic too, so you'll want to minimise the amount of stem that goes into your pot.

The berries are ripe when they're all black. Before this stage you will see some green and some red berries. To harvest, I recommend taking off the whole cluster of berries by snapping the stem off at the base. Picking the berries off individually will take a long time and will leave you with messy purple hands and not much in your basket! When you're home, pop the berry clusters into a Tupperware box and leave them in the freezer overnight.

In the morning you can simply pluck the berries off, or run through the delicate clusters with a fork. The berries will pop off into your bowl and none will be wasted due to accidental squashing!

Elderberry recipes

Elderberries have a tart, rich flavour and can be used to make sauces, jams and wines. They're best cooked fresh or from frozen; however, the berries can also be dried out to store throughout the year and made into delicious and immunity-boosting elderberry tea.

Plant lore, folk medicine & magic

The elder lives up to its reputation of giving us what we need when we need it, as the small black berries are filled with vitamins A and C and are high in antioxidants; they are traditionally used for their immune-boosting qualities. People would have traditionally made a syrup and had a tablespoon or two daily coming into the winter to help fight off colds and flu.

Remember, the elder is one of the most sacred trees in pagan and Celtic history, so it's important to ask the Elder Mother before taking any of her gifts.

Immunity-boosting elderberry syrup

Elderberries are used as an active ingredient in one of the most popular immunity-boosting medicines on the market. Yes, this is modern medicine I'm talking about! In general, folk medicines are ignored by modern medicine, perhaps because they cannot be patented. But elderberries are too powerful to ignore!

This elderberry syrup will do wonders for the immune system and tastes pretty special too. It can be taken by the tablespoon or used as an ingredient in cocktails and cakes.

MAKES APPROX. 400ML (14FL OZ)

800ml (3¼ cups) water
400g (14oz) fresh, frozen or dried elderberries
3 cinnamon sticks
Thumb-sized piece of fresh ginger, grated
1 lemon, unwaxed, sliced
1 large orange, unwaxed, sliced
20 cloves
1 star anise
170g (6oz) honey

1. Put all the ingredients, except the honey, into a large saucepan and bring to the boil.
2. Reduce the heat and simmer for 30 minutes, stirring regularly, until the mixture is thick and syrupy and reduced by at least half.
3. If you're using dried berries, add an extra 200ml (generous ¾ cup) water and simmer for an extra 10 minutes.
4. Remove from the heat and crush any remaining elderberries with the back of a fork.
5. Strain the mixture through a muslin cloth into a clean bowl. When the mixture is almost completely cool, stir through the honey.
6. Decant into a sterilised jar or bottle. Your syrup will last for up to 3 months and freezes very well for later use.

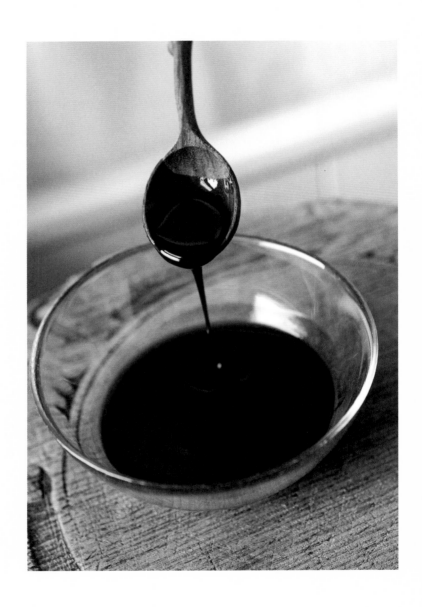

Elderberry and balsamic glaze

This deliciously dark and sticky glaze can be drizzled over salads, used as a dip for bread or in a sauce for rich meats and marinades. I use this all the time as a salad dressing for my workshops and always get such good feedback. I hope you enjoy it as much as my guests.

If you cannot find enough elderberries for your recipe, you can use a mix of elderberries and blackberries.

MAKES APPROX. 250ML (1 CUP)

150g (1 cup) frozen elderberries (if using fresh, reduce the cooking time by 10 minutes)
250ml (1 cup) good-quality balsamic vinegar
80ml (⅓ cup) maple syrup or good-quality honey

1. Put all the ingredients into a medium, heavy-based saucepan and bring to the boil.
2. Turn the heat down to a simmer and cook for about 20–30 minutes. Use the back of a fork to squash the elderberries down while they simmer.
3. When it's reduced by half, remove from the heat and allow to cool slightly. (The glaze will thicken as it cools so is best decanted when still slightly warm.)
4. Strain the mixture through a sieve, then pour into a sterilised jar or bottle and allow to cool completely before serving.
5. This glaze should last at least 3 weeks in the fridge and freezes well.

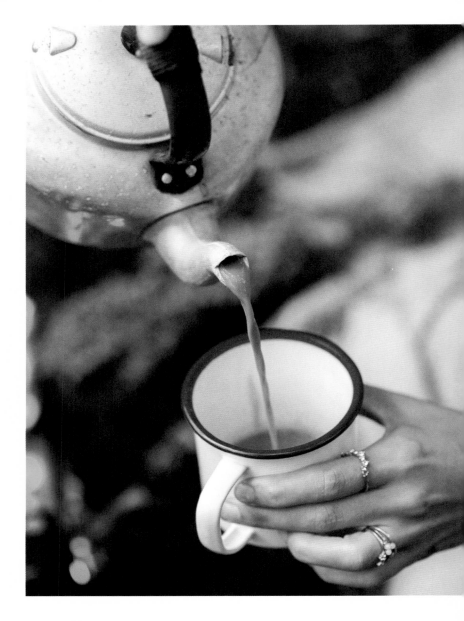

Autumn Self-care

Autumn is a fantastic time to draw the early nights around you like a blanket, get cosy and take some time to truly let go. Just like the trees drop their leaves, it's time for us to drop our expectations, our hurry and any past negativity we might be holding on to. It's a time to look inwards and allow slowness to take over.

Arts and crafts always come out of the woodwork for me during autumn. The crochet needles reappear, slow, dark hours are spent plaiting pastry for elaborate pies and autumn leaves are picked delicately from the ground and preserved in beeswax to make garlands and wall hangings.

It's such a beautiful time of year to let the outside in and using natural foraged elements in your crafting and decorating is sure to bring you more peace and joy in the coming long nights.

'Autumn is such a beautiful time of year to let the outside in.'

Autumn Rituals

Save seeds

Saving seeds is a wonderful thing to do for the environment. You can collect seeds from your favourite wild plants and give them a head start next spring, either by growing them in small pots and planting them up or simply by spreading them in your local meadows and hedgerows!

Remember to only take a small fraction of seeds so the plants can continue to grow where they are already thriving. Use a small paper bag to harvest your seeds and keep them over the winter until they're ready to use. There are plenty of YouTube tutorials on how to make origami envelopes and boxes, which you can do with recycled newspaper or pages from old books.

For some plants that hide their seeds away in closed buds, like evening primrose or poppies, the seed is best harvested by collecting dry flower heads and hanging them upside down in bundles with a paper bag wrapped around them to catch any falling seeds. When they're completely dry – after a week or two – you can cut open the flower buds and shake out the seeds.

If you'd like to make your seed-saving practice into more of a ritual, why not add a slip of paper to each envelope with an intention you'd like to grow alongside your wild plants? These could be personality traits or characteristics, like 'resilience' or 'strength', or they could be areas of your life you'd like to see development in, like 'a career I love' or relationships you'd like to see thrive, 'my connection with my partner' for example.

Host a harvest feast for autumn equinox

The autumn equinox occurs every year, sometime between September 21 and 24 in the northern hemisphere. Otherwise known as Mabon, named after the god of Welsh mythology, it aligns with modern-day harvest festivals and thanksgiving celebrations. It's historically a time to celebrate a successful harvest and the storing of food for the coming winter.

As the turning point between summer and autumn, it's an incredibly special time, when the night and the day are of equal length, and so we are thought to be in perfect balance. But from this day, the wheel will turn and we'll begin a transition to the darker half of the year. It's during this time that my knitted socks come out for a snuggle and the kitchen smells of pumpkin soup, roasting acorns and medicinal mushroom coffees.

Mabon is a time to give thanks for what you have had and what the earth has provided. Gather with family for an autumnal feast, or enjoy a quiet night of grateful reflection and some super-special acorn truffles (see page 204).

Releasing campfire ritual

There's nothing like a having a campfire as the nights get shorter. It's easy to tuck yourself away and not see friends but a campfire with loved ones is warming for the toes and the soul. Share hot drinks, toast marshmallows or make wild 'Nutella' damper bread on the fire. Sitting round a fire is, of course, ritual enough, but as autumn is a time for letting go why not take a moment to put this into action?

Think of the things that you'd like to let go of. They might be things from a long time ago, or perhaps from the last few months. They might be negative self-beliefs, things that you've done that you're not proud of and haven't forgiven yourself for, it might be negative thoughts towards another person, memories of something that someone has done to you or any number of other things. Releasing rituals such as the one below are perfect for autumn and it makes sense that they were traditionally practised around this time. If our negative thoughts are not released, there will be many a long, dark night to ruminate on them!

Letting negativity go can just be a case of deciding to let it go in the mind. But combining it with a physical action can strengthen this mental exercise. Letting something go is usually accompanied by a deep exhale, as if we're pushing that piece of negativity out with our breath. But to take it a step further, we can write down on a piece of paper all the things we no longer wish to hold and place it on the fire. If you aren't able to build a campfire, here's a simple way to do it with just a candle and a metal bowl:

1. Take a candle and a metal bowl, some matches, and a pen and a piece of paper. Light your candle and sit for a moment, taking a few deep breaths.
2. Bring to mind anything that might be holding you back and write it all out on your paper. Write until you feel lighter.
3. Now place your paper over the candle until it catches light, then transfer it to the metal bowl.
4. Envisage letting those things go as they burn and maybe even consider saying a few words along the lines of 'I release the belief that I am ...' 'I release the memory of ...'

After practising this ritual, take a few days to enjoy the lightness that you feel and then think about filling that gap with fresh creations, whether it be new, positive thoughts, plans for the future or physical crafty creations!

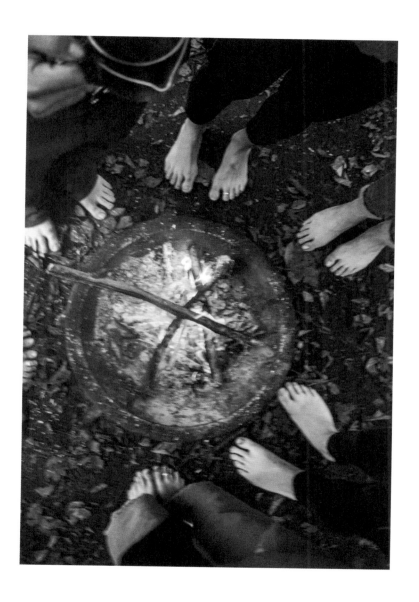

Winter

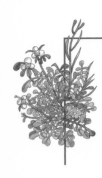

Shorter days have arrived, and the first signs of winter have started to appear. Still, silvery mists settle over the earth on chilly mornings, transforming familiar woodlands into places of mystery and magic. Robins seem to become more active and warble outside windows, proudly displaying their red chests, neatly matching the shining red berries displayed on now bare branches.

Eventually, a thin sheet of ice settles over the land, enhancing the sound of every footstep. Hurriedly crunching your way over the frozen ground to reach your warm destination is tempting, but if you stop to look, you'll see tiny pieces of art wherever you look. Frosty fallen leaves glitter in the winter sun and puddles crack into hundreds of glacial shards under your feet, stark and triangular, like mountain peaks.

When the abundance of autumn ends, the landscape can seem slightly bleak and it's easy to think we might have to hang up our boots until the arrival of spring. But worry not, there are still plenty of wonderful wild foods to be found in the wild spaces around you.

Winter is a time to regroup and regather, to reflect on the year behind and the year ahead. Enjoy the slow pace, revel in the festivities and conserve your energy for the coming year.

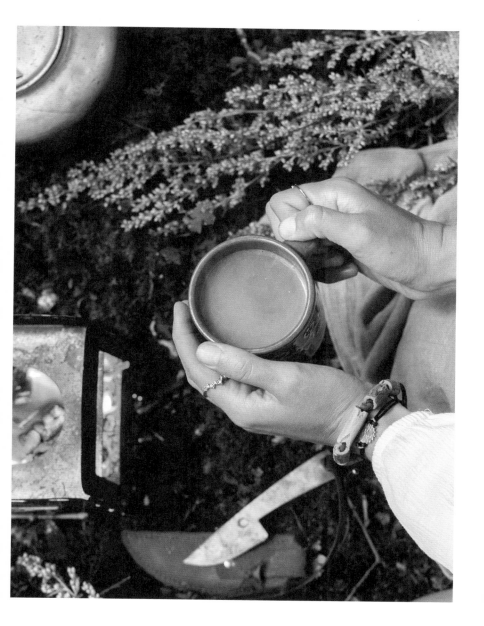

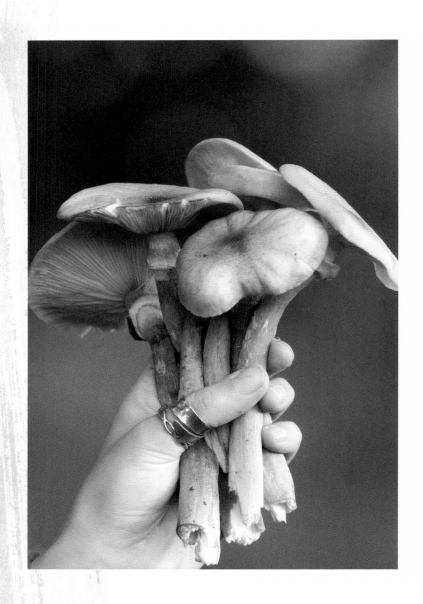

Foraging in Winter

Before the frosts come, some of our favourite greens make a reappearance; three-cornered leek and even wild garlic can be enjoyed again at this time of year. Mushroom season in its full autumnal glory has come to an end now but you may still find winter mushrooms such as jelly ears, turkey tails and velvet shanks. There aren't as many varieties on offer in winter, so it's time to hone your hunting skills and look out for those elusive, cold-loving mushrooms.

Discover little winter herbs like hairy bittercress, which can survive a full frosting and provides a source of vitamins even in the darkest of times. Seek out tall edible conifers which offer Christmassy pine needles for tea and cookies, and powerful medicinal mushrooms, waiting to be made into healing and nutritious broths and brews.

Although winter is a great time to forage, remember that it's as important as ever at this time of year that the last berries and nuts that might be lingering on bare branches are reserved for wildlife.

'In winter, plants retreat away from cold weather and take solace deep in the earth.'

Roots

We have a wonderful variety of edible roots to choose from in winter. They would have been an incredibly important food source for our ancestors and they're an amazingly fun and curious ingredient to harvest today. Roots are often forgotten about when it comes to wild foods, probably because we don't see them and they require a bit of digging to reveal themselves.

In winter, plants retreat away from cold weather and take solace deep in the earth. As their aerial parts (the fruits, leaves and stems) die away, they draw their energy – along with their sugars and nutrients – deep into their roots to conserve energy for warmer days. At this time, roots literally swell up, becoming larger and more nutrient-dense.

When it comes to harvesting roots, timing is key. You'll find that if you pick roots in the summer they'll be scrawny and fairly tasteless; but in winter, you'll have a wonderful, tasty ingredient. You do need to keep in mind that you'll need some aerial parts still alive to be able to find the root though. So for the best results, harvest at the very beginning of winter, before the plant has completely died away, or the very end of winter, when you can see a few green leaves to identify the plant. In colder climates, the best harvesting time might even be late autumn or early spring.

Also remember that you will need permission from the landowner to harvest wild roots and that by harvesting a root, you are ending the life of the plant. This is something we generally want to avoid; as foragers we want to have as little negative effect on the environment as possible. However, many edible roots are also garden weeds – plants that regularly and routinely get thrown on the compost heap. Pick from areas of abundance or gardens.

If you're looking to harvest large amounts of roots, for a dandelion and burdock beer perhaps, get in touch with a local gardener or allotmenteer friend; they may be able to supply you with a large amount of edible roots, if you ask!

Here is a list of wild roots for you to try:

Burdock	Wood avens
Dandelion	Bull thistle
Horseradish	Wild carrot

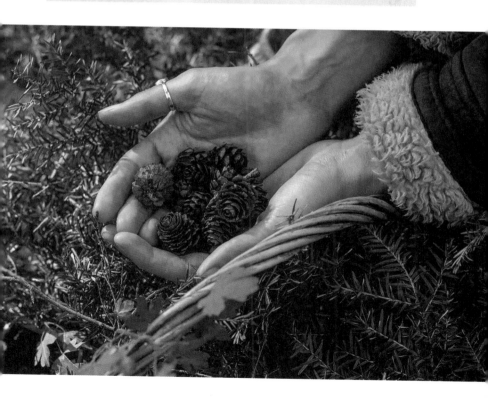

Jelly Ear Mushroom

[structure] Cup- or ear-shaped bracket mushrooms, becoming irregular and wobbly with age, with a jelly-like texture. Range from pink to orange to brownish in colour

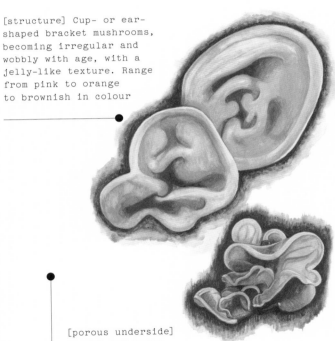

[porous underside] Smooth and shiny with wrinkles or creases, like the inside of an ear

[cap] Velvety to the touch; can grow up to 10cm (4in) across

Foraging notes

The jelly ear mushroom is a wonder to behold. It perfectly encapsulates the weird and wonderful world of fungi, with its squishy, jelly-like consistency and the way it dangles off trees like an old man's ear.

It has a long season and can be found throughout spring, autumn and winter, only dying back in the heat of the summer. Jelly ears are also particularly abundant and easy to find, growing almost exclusively on elder trees, although I've occasionally found them on holly. If you have a favourite stand of elder trees, start your hunt there.

Jelly ear mushroom recipes

After reading the introduction for this mushroom, or perhaps inquisitively prodding one you've seen on a nearby elder tree, you might not consider the kitchen to be a good place for the jelly ear mushroom. But don't be fooled by their odd appearance, they're a truly diverse and delicious ingredient!

They don't taste of much on their own, but they have an incredible ability to take on other flavours. Jelly ear mushrooms hold huge amounts of water and when dried, turn into thin little crisps. These crisps can be stored and rehydrated later; soaking them in warm water for 20 minutes will bring them back to their former glory, ready to be used in soups or risottos. However, if you want to inject some extra flavour into those little jellies, you can rehydrate them in a marinade of soy sauce, lime juice and ginger – perfect if you want to use them in a stir fry. Doing this transforms them from a tasteless but intriguing mushroom to the star of the show.

To prepare your mushroom, cut away any woody parts at the point it was connected to the tree and give it a good brush to remove any dirt. Use them fresh or dry as described in the recipes that follow.

Mushroom safety

Jelly ear mushrooms are very beginner-friendly. If you have a fungus that feels like jelly and is the shape of a cup or an ear, you're safe.

There are other types of jelly fungus, but none of them are known to be toxic. Most of them will simply look like splodges of jelly on a branch and none of them hold an ear-like shape. There are also some cup fungi which are similar in colour, but are decidedly brittle and in consistency, nothing like jelly.

'The jelly ear mushroom perfectly encapsulates the weird and wonderful world of fungi.'

Jelly ear mushroom dumplings

These dumplings are absolutely gorgeous – the filling is deeply mushroomy with lots of umami flavours and fragrant with wild winter herbs. You can fry or steam these dumplings, depending on what kind of texture you like. I've kept the recipe below nice and simple, but there are so many ways you can get more creative: try juicing some wild greens and adding the juice to the dumpling dough to make lovely green wrappers and, of course just playing with your wrapping style!

MAKES 20

165g (1⅓ cups) plain (all-purpose) flour
85g (1/3 cup) very hot water
1 tbsp coconut oil
150g (1 cup) jelly ear mushrooms
75g (½ cup) another mushroom of your choosing (velvet shanks or button mushrooms will work well), very finely chopped
2 tbsp soy sauce
½ tbsp white rice vinegar
1 tbsp honey

1. Tip the flour into a bowl and add the water gradually, mixing with chopsticks until all the flour is incorporated. Mix until a stiff dough is formed and then knead until smooth, about 10 minutes.

2. Return the dough to the bowl, cover and leave for about 1 hour at room temperature while you make the filling.

3. Heat the coconut oil in a frying pan and fry the mushrooms over a medium-high heat for 3 minutes, or until lightly browned. Add the soy sauce, white rice vinegar and honey and fry for a further 1 minute, then remove from the heat and stir through the herbs.

4. Cut the dough into 20 even pieces and roll them out into thin circles about 6cm (2½in) across. Put 1 level tablespoon of filling into the centre of each circle leaving a 1cm (½in) gap around the edges.

5. Gather up the outer edges of the circle to enclose the filling and pinch together to seal. Press down slightly so the dumplings have a flat bottom. Repeat until your filling has been used up.

6. Dip the bottom of each dumpling into water and then into the sesame seeds so the bottoms are coated with seeds.

Recipe continues over the page

15g (¼ cup) finely
  chopped mixed
  wild herbs (I
  used a mixture
  of ground ivy
  and cleavers.
  You could also
  use Thai basil or
  coriander/cilantro)
75g (½ cup)
  sesame seeds
Oil, for frying

7. Pour 1–2 tablespoons of oil into a high-sided frying pan with a lid and place over a high heat. Place the dumplings flat side down into the pan (you'll probably need to do this in two batches). Cook for 2 minutes until the dumplings are lightly browned on the base, then reduce the heat, add 60ml (¼ cup) water and cover tightly with a lid. Simmer gently for about 10 minutes, checking the water halfway through. Alternatively you can simply shallow-fry these for 4 minutes; carefully spoon hot oil over the tops of the dumplings so they are crispy and golden all over. Transfer to kitchen towel to drain away the excess oil before serving with your favourite dipping sauce.

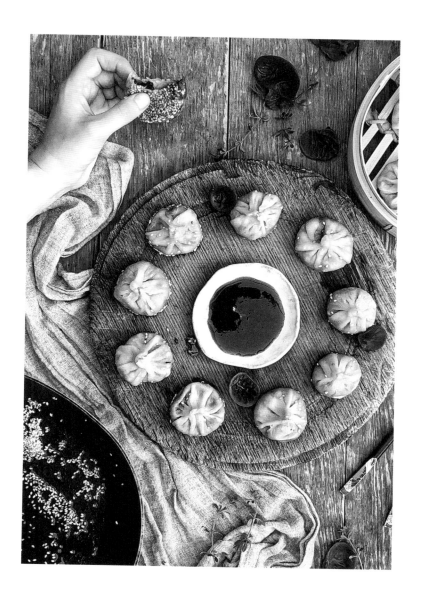

Jelly ear Jaffa cakes

If you're looking for a recipe to encourage your little ones to try some foraged mushrooms, look no further! Jelly ear mushrooms make the perfect substitute for the jelly layer in Jaffa cakes. If you're making these for adults, you can always soak your mushrooms in amaretto (my favourite option) or any other liquor of your choosing before dunking in chocolate.

I'm certainly not the first to have made jelly ear Jaffa cakes; I heard about them from my friend Richard Mawby (@foragefrolics), and while the origin of these jelly ear Jaffa cakes is hard to pin down, Fergus Drennan (@Fergustheforager) is a likely candidate for inventor! Here's my recipe for them.

MAKES 20

20 jelly ear mushrooms, as close to 4cm (1½in) across as you can find
240ml (1 cup) smooth orange juice
100g (scant 1 cup) self-raising flour
60g (2oz) caster (superfine) sugar
100ml (3½fl oz) milk (or non-dairy milk)
50ml (2fl oz) sunflower oil
1 tsp vanilla extract
150g (5oz) chocolate of your choice (I like using 70% dark chocolate, but kids might prefer milk chocolate)

1. Preheat the oven to its lowest setting. Lay your jelly ear mushrooms out on a baking tray and place them in the oven for 2 hours. This will partially dry the jelly ear mushrooms and they should be not completely dehydrated. Set aside to cool.

2. Add the mushrooms to a bowl, pour over the orange juice, then cover and allow to rehydrate overnight (warming the orange juice slightly can help with the rehydrating process).

3. The following day, drain the mushrooms and leave them to air-dry while you make the cakes.

4. Preheat the oven to 180°C/350°F/gas 4 and line and grease a 20cm (8in) square cake tin.

5. Sift the flour and sugar into a bowl, then add the milk, oil and vanilla extract and stir until combined.

6. Pour into the cake tin and bake for 25–30 minutes, or until a wooden skewer comes out clean and the sponge springs back when pressed. Transfer the cake to a wire rack and allow to cool.

7. Meanwhile, melt the chocolate: break it into pieces and add to a heatproof bowl set over a pan of just simmering water (or use a microwave).

Strips of orange zest
or candied orange
peel, to decorate

8. When the sponge has cooled, use a round cutter or a shot glass measuring roughly 4cm (1½in) across to cut out 20 cake rounds.

9. Drape a jelly ear mushroom over each cake round and then dip into the melted chocolate. Transfer to a sheet of baking paper and leave to set at room temperature. Decorate with orange zest or candied peel.

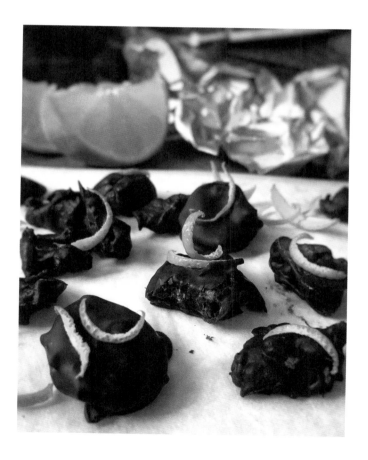

Sloe

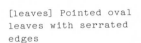

[leaves] Pointed oval
leaves with serrated
edges

[bark and
branch]
Hedgerow shrub
or tree with
inch-long
thorns. New
growth has a
purple tint

[flowers] White
blossom in spring

[fruit] Round,
dark purple to
black fruit with
a dusty, light
blue coating and
a stone in the
centre

Foraging notes

If you've never tried a sloe straight from the tree, I need you to do so with immediate effect. I promise the result will be hilarious! They have a big stone in the middle but the fleshy fruit around the stone is incredibly sour and takes all the moisture out of your mouth. I spent many a happy childhood walk trying to offer them up as 'wild blueberries' for the sheer joy of watching people's reactions on biting into the flesh.

Sloes grow from the blackthorn, which is a very common hedgerow tree. They are the great-grandmother of our modern-day, cultivated garden plums and played a vital role in our history as hunter-gatherers. Stones from sloes have been found in archaeological sites from the Mesolithic and Iron Age periods, suggesting they were part of early man's diet. If you've taken my earlier advice and tried a sloe, this is sure to come as a shock: imagine a lunch of sloes!

You'll know the sloes are ready to harvest when they have a dusty coating that can be rubbed off and are slightly squishy to the touch. If they're very hard, leave them for a few more weeks or pop them in the freezer overnight. It's the 'first frost' which makes them squishy and sweet; as the berry freezes the juice inside expands and stretches the skin. Popping them in the freezer mimics this natural sweetening process. They're usually perfect between November and December.

Sloe recipes

I have found that sloe gin is the only thing that can completely remove the sourness and the capacity to dry out the mouth that comes with sloes. Of course, I'm not complaining, you can't do much better than sloe gin in my opinion. It's the perfect winter drink, simply served as it is in a small glass, but it can be used to make plenty of other things! Sloe gin can be the star ingredient in delicious cocktails, sponge puddings, jellies, ice creams, cakes and tarts.

Sloes can also be used in chutneys and jams with success, but use with other fruits and keep the proportion of sloes small.

Plant lore, folk medicine & magic

With such a long history, it's no surprise that a wealth of folklore – or treelore – surrounds this magical plant. Because it is one of the fruits that remain on the branches throughout the winter, it would have been a staple and a sign of the dark times, where the pains of hunger would have been real. A long, hard winter has been referred to throughout history as a 'Blackthorn Winter' and in Scottish folk tales, winter begins when the Cailleach (the goddess of winter) strikes the ground with her blackthorn staff.

The tree itself is known as the Dark Crone of the Woods, the keeper of dark magic and secrets, with strong links to witches who perform dark magic. In British folklore, a witch would use a blackthorn to pierce a doll who would represent a person to be cursed. In south Devon folklore, witches were said to carry blackthorn walking sticks, with which they caused much local mischief. And in the witch burnings, the burners, in an ironic twist, would burn the witches on blackthorn pyres.

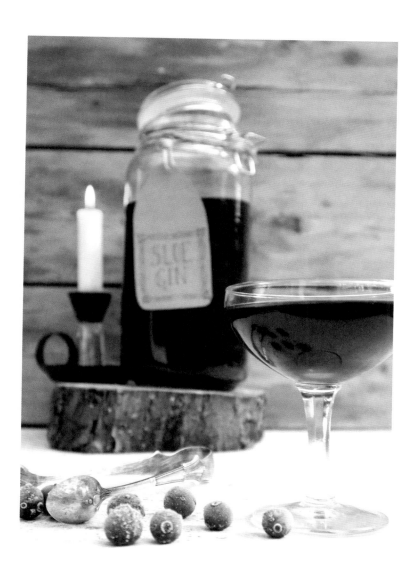

Perfect sloe gin

Here's my go-to recipe for perfect sloe gin. You'll see it doesn't include any sugar —sloes have loads of natural sugars and adding more can inhibit the flow of fruit into the alcohol. I think the taste is much better and purer without and you can always add some simple sugar syrup when it's done if you prefer it sweeter.

I tend to make my gin in November and leave it for a full year until the following Christmas. You'll have to wait until you crack it open, but then some things are worth waiting for – just remember to make another batch so you always have one in rotation!

500g (1lb 2oz) sloes
1 cinnamon stick
    (optional)
5 cloves (optional)
2 star anise
    (optional)
700ml (2¾ cups) gin

1. Harvest your sloes and put them in the freezer overnight (see page 257).
2. In the morning, defrost the sloes for a minimum of 3 hours and then add them to a 2-litre (3½-pint) sterilised jar or bottle with a tight-fitting lid. Add the spices if you're using them.
3. Top up the jar with gin, close and shake vigorously,
4. Shake the jar every day for 5 days and then leave somewhere cool and dark for a minimum of 6 months.
5. When it's ready to drink, you can pour out some of the gin whenever you'd like a tot (you can't over-brew sloe gin so don't worry about straining out the sloes). Alternatively, decant into smaller bottles to gift to your loved ones.

Sloe and Fizzy

Straight sloe gin goes down far too easily around the fire on winter nights! These sloe gin fizzys are the perfect way to make it last. Refreshing, tangy with a dark, fruit kick, these will make those winter nights much warmer.

45ml (1½ oz) sloe gin
30ml (1 oz) freshly squeezed lemon juice
30ml (1 oz) rosehip, elderberry or sloe syrup
Frozen sloes
Club soda or plain seltzer water and edible seasonal sprigs, to garnish

1. To a cocktail shaker or glass jar, add the sloe gin, lemon juice and syrup then top up with ice. Shake until chilled.
2. Fill a tall glass with ice and a few frozen sloes, and strain the contents of your cocktail shaker or glass jar into the glass.
3. Top up with Club soda or plain seltzer water and garnish!

The Dark Crone

This cocktail is based on Lottie Muir's blackberry and lilac cobbler from her amazing book *Wild Cocktails*. We made them a few years ago and fell deeply in love! We've been playing around with our own version ever since. These short, punchy little cocktails are an incredible mix of smoky whiskey and dark fruits.

7-10 blackberries (save a few for garnish)
1 tsp (5ml) blackcurrant cassis
45ml (1½ oz) sloe gin
30ml (1 oz) whiskey
15ml (½ oz) freshly squeezed lemon juice
15ml (½ oz) elderberry syrup

1. Add the blackberries (reserving 2 or 3 to garnish) and the cassis to a cocktail shaker or glass jar and muddle or 'smoosh' with a muddler or the end of a rolling pin.
2. Add the other ingredients and shake well until combined.
3. Fill a short glass with crushed ice and pour the contents of your cocktail shaker over the ice. Garnish with your blackberries and any seasonal edible wildflowers you fancy.

Rosehip

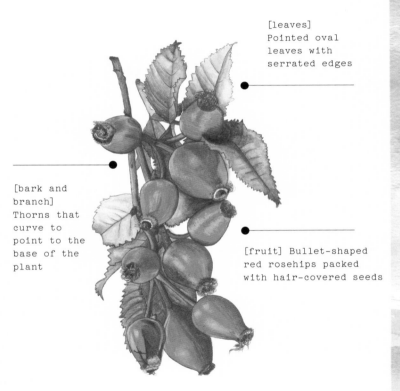

[leaves]
Pointed oval
leaves with
serrated edges

[bark and
branch]
Thorns that
curve to
point to the
base of the
plant

[fruit] Bullet-shaped
red rosehips packed
with hair-covered seeds

[flowers] Five-
petalled pink
flowers

Foraging notes

When the temperature drops and the last petals fall from the roses, the hips begin to ripen. Shining red rosehips are already like jewels in the hedgerows and with a little love, they make wonderful syrups and sweets!

All rosehips are edible, whether they are wild dog roses or garden roses, so you may well find rosehips in your own garden. Rosehips are red berries, packed full of tiny seeds covered in hairs. Wild rosehips tend to have an elongated, bullet shape, whereas garden rosehips may be fatter and rounder. If you're foraging in the wild, look for bullet-shaped berries on thorny branches to avoid confusing these with anything that is not edible.

Rosehip recipes

When cooking with rosehips you want the sweet red flesh as that's where the goodness is. It's important that none of the seeds or hairs that cover the seeds make their way into the finished product. The hairs are incredibly itchy (in fact they used to be used as itching powder) and they can also irritate the stomach, so they shouldn't be consumed.

Taking out the seeds can be done at the beginning of the process or the end. You can either cut each rosehip in half and scoop out the seeds and hairs with a small spoon (this is very time-consuming but necessary if you want to keep the form of the hips). Or, if you're making syrup or jam, you can strain your finished product several times through a muslin cloth before using and eating.

Like most wild berries, rosehips are sweetest after the first frost. You can substitute them in the elderberry syrup recipe on page 231: simply blend the rosehips and water in a blender to make a slurry before you start and repeat the step where you strain through a muslin cloth twice, to ensure you've removed all the scratchy hairs.

Plant lore, folk medicine & magic

Rosehips were such a valuable food source in times gone by, because of their ridiculously high levels of vitamin C – almost 13 times higher than oranges. They also have powerful anti-inflammatory qualities, which studies show may help people with heart disease and even arthritis. Because of this, traditional rosehip syrup was a well-known medicine/sweet treat. In fact, during the Second World War, the valued hips were gathered by schools, Boy Scouts and Girl Guides and the Women's Institutes, taken to local councils and made into syrup to ward off malnutrition.

In English folklore, a particularly fat rosehip, bursting with seeds, was thought to be a lucky token that would bring the owner great wealth and heightened fertility.

Candied rosehips

Candied rosehips make the perfect Christmas gift; boiled and rolled in sugar, they look like sparkling red gems and taste superb, with a flavour that is jammy, floral and sweet. They can be used in a number of ways: eat like sweets straight from the jar, stir into mince pie or Christmas cake recipes, or simply simmer in a saucepan with water to make rosehip syrup or jam. Heaven.

**MAKES APPROX.
1 FULL JAR**

400g (14oz) hard rosehips, (picked before the first frost)
120ml (½ cup) water
300g (1½ cups) granulated sugar

1. First process your rosehips. Cut them open lengthways (this part may be tricky, so mind your fingers) and use a small spoon to thoroughly remove all the seeds and hairs from inside. Wash the emptied rosehips thoroughly and allow to dry.
2. Pour the water and 100g (½ cup) of the sugar into a medium saucepan. Bring to the boil, then reduce the heat and let it simmer over a low heat for 3 minutes.
3. Stir in the rosehips until they are fully coated in the sugar solution, then remove from the heat and continue to stir for 1 minute.
4. Remove the rosehips with a slotted spoon and transfer to a baking sheet lined with baking paper. Allow to partially dry for around 1 hour.
5. Put the remaining sugar into a shallow bowl and roll the almost-dry rosehips in the sugar until coated. Transfer to a warm, dry place and allow to dry completely overnight. In the morning, the rosehips can be placed in an airtight container.
6. These candied rosehips will last for at least 3 months.

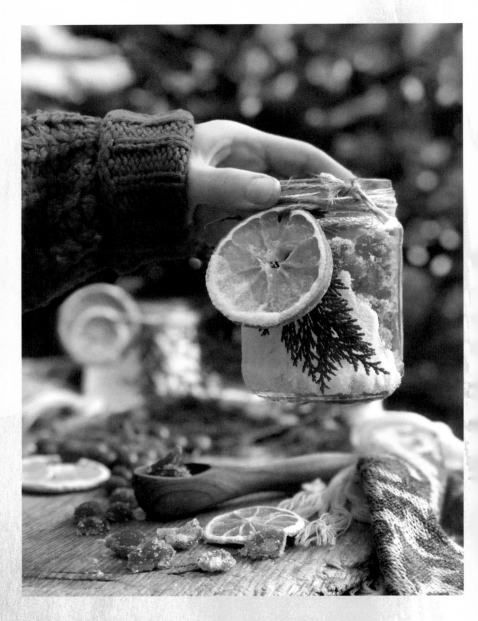

Candied rosehip Florentines

This Florentine recipe is adapted from one we use every Christmas, from the wonderful Mary Berry. It's the perfect way to use your candied rosehips and makes for the most special of biscuits. If you're planning on gifting someone a jar of candied rosehips this Christmas, you could write out this recipe for them to try!

MAKES 10

30g (1oz) butter
30g (1oz)
   demerara sugar
30g (1oz)
   golden syrup
30g (⅓oz) plain
   (all-purpose) flour
20g (¾oz) dried
   cranberries,
   finely chopped
30g (1oz) candied
   rosehips (see
   page 265), finely
   chopped
15g (½oz) almonds,
   finely chopped
15g (½oz) hazelnuts,
   finely chopped
200g (7oz) dark
   chocolate,
   roughly chopped

1. Preheat the oven to 180°C/350°F/gas 4 and line a couple of baking trays with baking paper.
2. Melt the butter, sugar and syrup in a saucepan over a low heat.
3. Remove from the heat and add the rest of the ingredients, except the chocolate. Stir until all the ingredients are combined.
4. Spoon out teaspoons of the mixture on to each baking tray, leaving plenty of space between each spoonful. You should get five on each tray.
5. Bake for 8 minutes, or until golden brown. Remove from the oven and allow to cool.
6. Melt the chocolate: put the chocolate pieces into heatproof bowl and set over a saucepan of just simmering water, making sure the base of the bowl doesn't touch the water. Stir until melted. Alternatively, melt in the microwave in short bursts, stirring the chocolate between each burst.
7. Dip the bottom of each Florentine into the melted chocolate. At this point you can make a zigzag pattern with a fork if you'd like.
8. Transfer the Florentines to a plate and allow to cool completely upside down until the chocolate is set.

Dandelion Root

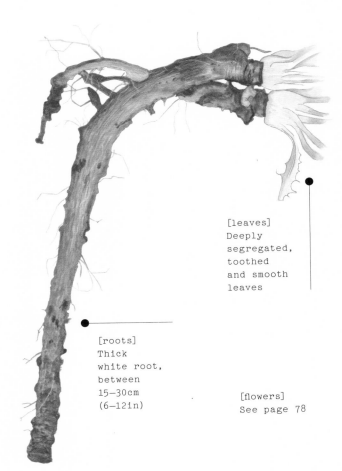

[leaves]
Deeply
segregated,
toothed
and smooth
leaves

[roots]
Thick
white root,
between
15—30cm
(6—121n)

[flowers]
See page 78

Foraging notes

Dandelion root is an abundant root vegetable and a powerhouse of nutrition. It's also incredibly fun to dig up.

It's so easy to get your hands on a good harvest of dandelion roots. If you don't have any in your garden, why not put up a post on social media and see if anyone wants you to come and dig up theirs? I bet you'll have more than a few offers! If you don't fancy doing the hard work yourself, ask a friend with a garden or allotment if you can have theirs next time they have a weeding session.

When you're harvesting dandelions make sure to leave some in your garden or local wild space as they actually do quite important work to improve the soil.

Dandelion root recipes

Dandelion root can be used like any other root vegetable but it is incredibly bitter. I've chopped it up fresh and had it in stews but I did have to keep reminding myself how good for me it was in order to finish the bowl!

For the best dandelion dishes, either make something that should be bitter, like coffee or even bitters to use in cocktails, or make something sweet so the flavour balances out. Fermenting dandelion root also removes a lot of the bitterness so you can grate it into homemade sauerkraut. It's also great for dandelion and burdock drinks.

Plant lore, folk medicine & magic

Dandelion root has long been used in Chinese and Native American medicine for a range of ailments, including stomach and liver problems and skin complaints.

Dandelion is a symbol for positive change, transformation and community. This is because the dandelion's long taproot burrows deep into the earth, through hard and rocky areas that other plants cannot access. It breaks up the ground, encouraging the activity of earthworms, which bring buried nutrients to the soil surface for other plants to benefit from.

'Dandelion is a symbol for positive change, transformation and community.'

Dandelion latte

Dandelion latte is a marvel. The bitterness of the root lends itself wonderfully to coffee and because it's caffeine free, it makes the perfect cosy bedtime drink for coffee lovers. For this recipe you'll need to dry and then powder your dandelion root. These instructions can be used to dry any edible root.

MAKES 2 CUPS

Handful of
  dandelion roots
500ml (2 cups)
  milk of choice
½ tsp ground
  cinnamon
  (optional)
Maple syrup or
  honey, to taste

1. Preheat the oven to its lowest setting 90°C/195°F/gas ¼, unless you have a dehydrator.

2. Harvest your roots, chop off the leaves and stems and put them on the compost heap. Wash your roots with warm water, removing any mud. You'll only need a small amount of dried dandelion powder for this recipe but it's worth preparing a few roots to store for future use in an airtight jar. They will last for up to a year and are best ground just before use for maximum nutrient density and flavour.

3. Cut the dandelion root into thin, even strips roughly 5cm (2in) long and 2cm (¾in) across. Spread out on a baking tray in a single layer and bake for around 4 hours, stirring and turning occasionally until completely dry. Alternatively you can dry out the roots in a dehydrator. Allow the dried roots to cool completely.

4. Grind the roots like regular coffee beans, or powder them in a spice grinder or pestle and mortar. You'll want to grind them to as fine a powder as possible.

5. Warm the milk in a small saucepan so it's hot but not boiling. Whisk in 2 tablespoons of your fine dandelion root powder. Warm for another 2 minutes. If you have not managed to grind your dandelion to a fine enough powder, at this point you should pass it through a muslin cloth to remove any large pieces of dandelion. Then return to the pan.

6. Whisk in the ground cinnamon, if using. Sweeten to taste with maple syrup or honey and froth with a milk frother, if you have one.

Dandelion coffee yule log

This yule log will be the star of the show at your Christmas table. You could replace the dandelion root powder with a powder made from dried turkey tail, or even add some wood avens root powder for some wild spice!

MAKES 12 SLICES

For the sponge
2 tbsp
  self-raising flour
50g (½ cup)
  cocoa powder
Pinch of salt
5 large eggs,
  separated
130g (⅔ cup)
  granulated sugar
½ tsp vanilla extract
2 tbsp melted butter
2 tbsp icing
  (confectioner's)
  sugar

For the filling
250ml (1 cup)
  whipping cream
3 tbsp dandelion root
  powder (see page
  271), dissolved in
  ½ tbsp water
65g (½ cup) icing
  (confectioner's)
  sugar

1. Preheat the oven to 200°C/400°F/gas 6. Line and grease a 45 x 33cm (18 x 13in) Swiss roll tin with baking paper.

2. Sift the flour, cocoa powder and salt together in a bowl and whisk together. Add the eggs and sugar to the bowl of a stand mixer and mix on medium speed until very light and fluffy. Add the dry ingredients and the vanilla extract and stir until just combined. Pour in the melted butter and mix again.

3. Pour the mixture into the lined tin and bake for 8–10 minutes, or until a skewer comes out clean and the sponge springs back when pressed. Allow to cool in the tin for 5 minutes.

4. Liberally sprinkle a clean tea towel with half of the icing sugar, then flip the cake on to the top and sprinkle the other side with the remaining icing sugar. Roll the cake up in the towel starting at one of the short sides. Leave in the towel for 30 minutes.

5. Meanwhile, make the filling. Whip the cream to soft peaks, then fold in the dandelion root mixture and icing sugar. Now make the buttercream: add all the ingredients to a bowl and use a hand-held whisk to beat together until smooth and combined.

For the buttercream
75g (3oz) butter,
   softened
250g (2 cups) icing
   (confectioner's)
   sugar
30g (⅓ cup) cocoa
   powder
1 tbsp dandelion
   root powder (see
   page 271),
   dissolved in
   ½ tbsp water
1 tsp vanilla extract
3 tbsp milk

6. To assemble the yule log, unroll the now-cooled sponge from the tea towel. Spread the filling over the sponge, taking the cream almost to the edges. Roll up the sponge and position the log seam side down. Use a palette knife to spread the buttercream over the top and sides of the log.

7. Decorate with some candied rosehips (see page 265) and meringue mushrooms, if you like.

Hairy Bittercress

[flowers]
Small flowers
with four
white petals

[seeds] Long
seed pods,
similar to
pea pods

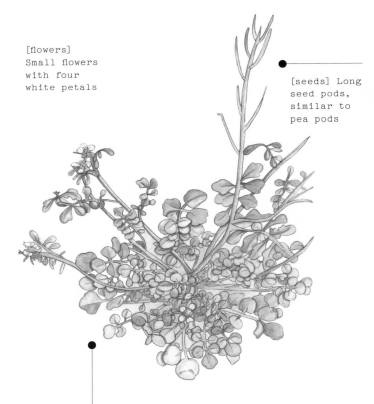

[leaves] Low-lying rosette of stems.
Each stem has an opposite pair of
leaves and one larger leaf at the
end of the stem

Foraging notes

Hairy bittercress is a delicious winter green that is neither hairy not bitter. It's from the mustard family and is perfectly crisp and smooth, much like the bagged salad leaves you find in supermarkets. It has a peppery taste that makes for a flavoursome salad.

Hairy bittercress is another plant with a wealth of common names, hoary bittercress, lamb's cress, land cress and spring cress to name a few, signifying it was an important plant for people in England throughout history.

Be careful when you harvest hairy bittercress because it's very easy to uproot it accidentally and unnecessarily. It's best to harvest it by taking a few stems from each plant. If it's found in abundance, use scissors to carefully snip off a few whole heads.

Hairy bittercress recipes

Hairy bittercress leaves are a brilliant base for a winter salad, a great addition to sandwiches and make a lovely garnish. They can also be used like spinach, as a nutritious addition to many dishes. Add it to a dish for the last few minutes if you intend to cook with it.

Plant lore, folk medicine & magic

Hairy bittercress is packed full of vitamins A and C, calcium and magnesium. In Saxon folklore, hairy bittercress was thought to draw out venom and poison. It would be poulticed and applied to bites to clean the wound and bring pain relief.

Forager's Welsh rarebit

This is my go-to recipe when I have a few big handfuls of wild herbs. It really does work with most wild herbs – cleavers, nettles or ground ivy to name a few – but the pepperiness of hairy bittercress works perfectly here. A herby, vibrant, rich and cheesy forager's Welsh rarebit, this recipe would work beautifully with lots of garden herbs too – basil, oregano, chives or nasturtiums would be dreamy!

MAKES 3 SLICES

3 slices of white bread
5 heads of hairy bittercress
Small handful of another wild green of your choice
2 tbsp good-quality olive oil
20g (¾oz) butter
1 tbsp plain (all-purpose) flour
170ml (⅔ cup) milk
½ tbsp Dijon mustard
Large handful of grated mature Cheddar cheese (about 40g/1½oz)
Salt and freshly ground black pepper

1. Lightly toast the slices of bread.
2. Roughly chop the bittercress and other wild greens, then pop into a food processor with the olive oil and blend until you have a fairly smooth paste.
3. Melt the butter in a saucepan, then add the flour and stir over a medium heat for a minute or two. Slowly add the milk, stirring all the time, until you have a white sauce. Add the mustard and reduce over a low-medium heat until the sauce begins to thicken. Add the grated cheese, then taste and season with salt and pepper.
4. Preheat the grill to high.
5. Thinly spread the herb paste over your toast and then spoon over your cheese sauce. Pop under the grill and wait until your sauce is bubbling and brown. Remove from the heat and serve immediately.

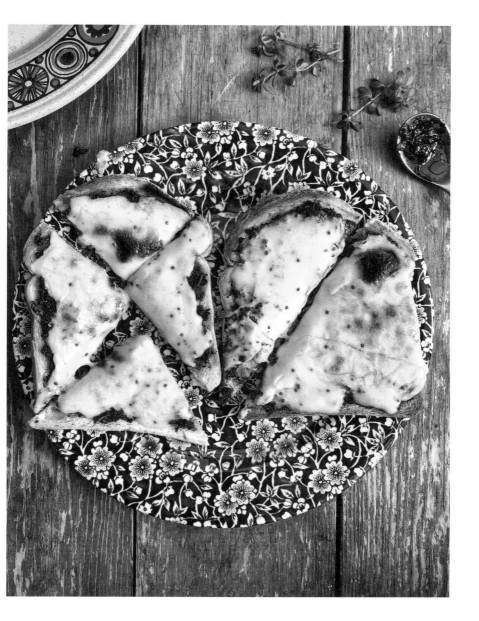

Winter Self-care

Winter is a time for death and rebirth. Last year's sun will run its course and die to make way for the next year's sun, yet to give us longer days and radiate its warmth and light. Think about the elements or habits in your life that you're ready to let go of and the new ones you want to birth for the coming year.

Winter Rituals

Embrace the solstice spirit and give gifts in celebration and love. It might be a gift to yourself, for example the gift of a day spent alone, really listening to your thoughts, dreams and desires. It might be a gift to a loved one, a poem or a word of thanks for their presence in the previous year. Or maybe a gift to those less fortunate or to the earth itself.

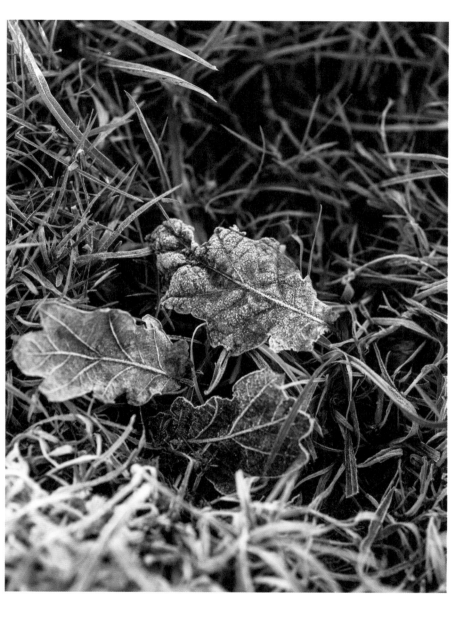

Celebrating Christmas and the winter solstice

The day of the winter solstice, which usually falls on 21 December, is the shortest day of the year. It is the depth of the winter and the darkest time. But although those short, dark days can seem eternal, with the darkness comes the promise of light. From today onwards, the darkness will retreat, and lighter, brighter days are ahead. The perfect cause for celebration!

Like the summer solstice, this was an incredibly important day for our hunter-gatherer ancestors.

People gathered and meats, fermented dairy products and mead were consumed in great quantities; pieces of gold jewellery have been discovered dating back to the same time, suggesting they were wearing their finest clothes or perhaps exchanging gifts.

Winter solstice celebrations slowly transformed into Christmas celebrations as the cultural tide turned. Where the returning of the sun was once celebrated, the coming of the 'son' of God became the focus of our festivities, but many of the themes and symbols carried over.

For me, winter solstice, Christmas and New Year roll into one happy celebration – we give gifts, share feasts and make plans and promises for the year ahead. I love giving edible gifts: hot, spiced caramelised nuts, candied rosehips, chocolate bark and meringue mushrooms are just some ideas.

Make wild Christmas gift jars

If you're making wild gifts this year, like meringue mushrooms or candied rosehips, you'll need something beautiful to present them in. Why not try making snowy Christmas jars by mixing a tablespoon of flour and water together to make a glue, then brushing this mixture to the outside of your sterilised jar before sprinkling with salt? Set aside to dry for a couple of hours and you'll have lovely wintry jars to give your gifts in (see photo on page 266). You can add extra decoration with lengths of twine, conifer sprigs and slices of dried orange.

Make a pine cone birdfeeder

January and February can be hungry months for our wildlife so it's important that we leave the last wild fruits and nuts for the birds, but also leave some healthy treats out for them too! These foraged pine cone birdfeeders provide much needed nutrition for tits, starlings, sparrows and plenty of other small feathered friends.

To make your birdfeeders, simply wrap some twine around a pine cone, tie in tightly and make a long loop so you will be able to hang the finished product from branches. Smother peanut butter generously over the pine cone and then roll in your birdseed (this will be messy!). Head outside to hang the pine cone up and enjoy keeping an eye on them to see who pays a visit.

You don't have to have a garden to hang birdfeeders; take a few in a Tupperware box on your walk and leave them in trees where you can hear birdsong

Attend a wassail

Wassail is one of my favourite celebrations of the year. It's decidedly odd, downright bizarre and utterly hilarious in most cases!

Wassail usually takes place in January, traditionally on the Twelfth Night and the word can be applied to both the ceremony and a traditional drink (a hot spiced cider) which is served at the ceremony. A wassail is a chance to wish good health to neighbours, animals and crops with the cider, which is either drunk or sprinkled over the ground. As well as being about blessing the apple trees, ceremonies also involve driving away any bad spirits that may try to hamper a good harvest.

I highly recommend trying to attend a wassail ceremony; you should be able to find one with through a quick google search.

If you'd rather, though, you can always hold a personal wassail for yourself. Start by making your favourite drink. Think about what herbs or flavours resonate with you, what you enjoy and what makes you feel good. Remember you're thanking your body with this gift.

Sit down and think about what actions or behaviours have led to bounty during the previous year. Maybe you made time for regular exercise, maybe you took a class to learn something new or maybe you enjoyed more time for stillness and reflection.

With each sip of your drink, thank yourself for those actions. Imagine drinking in the bounty they have produced and imagine the cycle repeating.

'A wassail is a chance to wish good health to neighbours, animals and crops.'

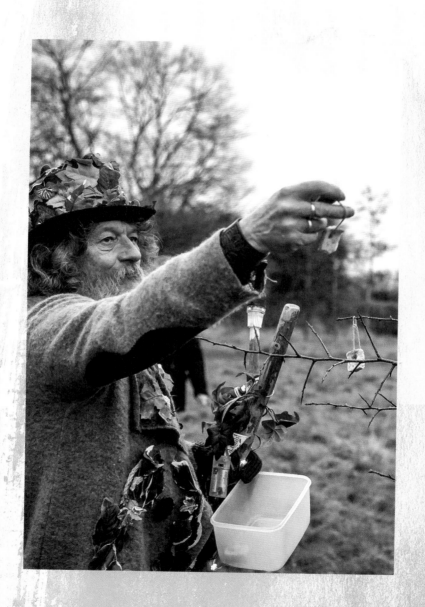

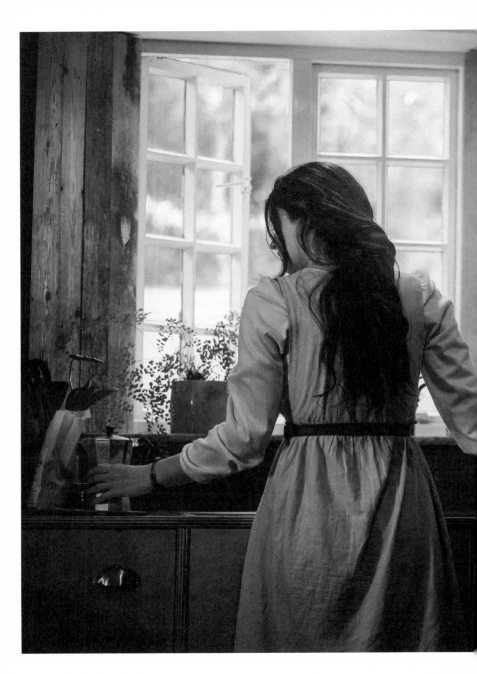

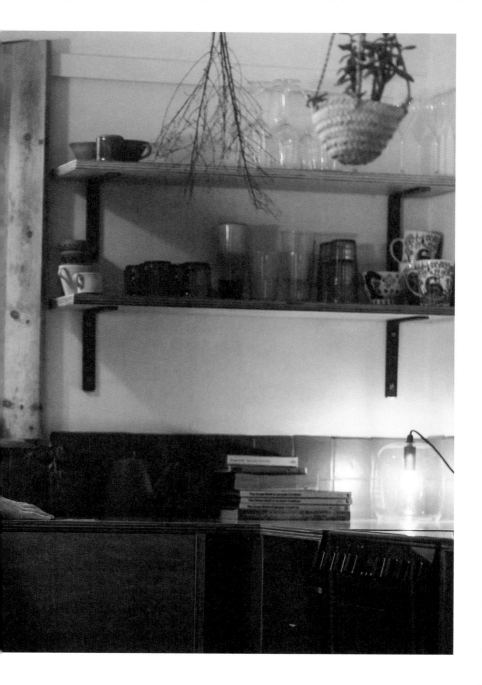

Acknowledgements

I would like to thank the foraging community at large. The amazing online and real-world community of people touched by the magic of wild plants is a constant source of knowledge, ideas and fun! I have named direct sources of inspiration where possible but I'm sure there are many indirect sources too. As is the way of inspiration, it often blooms from a forgotten root, buried deep in the mind, something once read, seen or heard about.

I'd also like to thank the wonderful people who have contributed photos to this book. Josh (@joshwaar), Toni (@cuttlebone.co.uk), Alice (@shot_by_alice), Sam (@adriftvisuals), Marina (@dfnstudios) for the pictures of me frolicking in nature with my basket, and Nigel Cull (@Nigelcull) for the merry wassail photos. Thank you for helping me capture the magic.

Index of herbs, wildflowers and mushrooms

1

Ebury Press, an imprint of Ebury Publishing
20 Vauxhall Bridge Road,
London SW1V 2SA

Ebury Press is part of the Penguin Random House group of companies
whose addresses can be found at global.penguinrandomhouse.com

 Penguin
Random House
UK

Text © Fern Freud 2023
Photography © Fern Freud, Josh Ryall, Cuttlebone Photography,
Alice Greenfield, DFN Studios and Nigel Cull 2023
Illustrations © Laura Tindorf 2023

Fern Freud has asserted her right to be identified as the author of this
Work in accordance with the Copyright, Designs and Patents Act 1988

First published by Ebury Press in 2023

www.penguin.co.uk

A CIP catalogue record for this book is available from the British Library

ISBN 9781529198218

Photography: Fern Freud, Josh Ryall, Cuttlebone Photography,
Alice Greenfield, DFN Studios and Nigel Cull
Design: Studio Polka
Illustrations: Laura Tindorf
Colour reproduction: Altaimage London Ltd

Printed and bound in China by C&C Offset Printing Co., Ltd

The authorised representative in the EEA is Penguin Random House Ireland,
Morrison Chambers, 32 Nassau Street, Dublin D02 YH68.

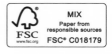

Penguin Random House is committed to a sustainable future for our business,
our readers and our planet. This book is made from Forest Stewardship
Council® certified paper.